2024 LOW GLYCEMIC INDEX AND LOAD DIABETES DIET

SIMPLE SCIENCE-BASED MEAL PLANS WITH GI, GL & CARB COUNTER, DIABETES-FRIENDLY FOOD COUNTER, AND COMPREHENSIVE FOOD LISTS

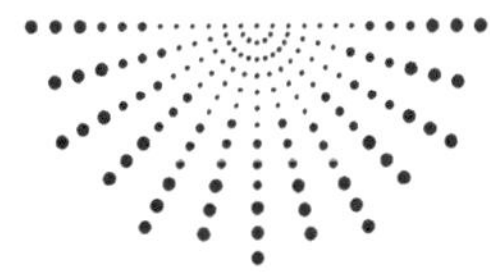

DR. H. MAHER

ISBN: 9798325568985

Medical Disclaimer:

Accuracy and Diligence:

The author and publisher of "2024 Low Glycemic Index & Load Diabetes Diet" have made every effort to ensure the accuracy and completeness of the information provided within this publication. Extensive research and careful consideration have been employed to present data and insights that reflect the latest and most relevant information available up to the date of publication.

Use of Up-to-Date Information:

This book incorporates the latest data and insights available in the field of nutrition and diabetes management at the time of writing. The author and publisher are committed to using the most current and scientifically validated information to support the recommendations and advice provided herein.

General Information:

The dieting and nutritional guidance offered in this book is intended for informational purposes only and does not constitute medical advice, diagnosis, treatment, or any other professional healthcare advice. Due to the unique nature of each individual's health conditions and nutritional needs, the content may not be appropriate for everyone.

Consultation with Healthcare Professionals:

It is crucial for readers to consult with their physician or another qualified healthcare professional before initiating any new dieting, weight loss, or exercise program, especially those with pre-existing health conditions, those under medical treatment, or individuals with specific dietary needs and restrictions. Continuous supervision by a healthcare provider is recommended to ensure the safety and appropriateness of any dietary and lifestyle changes made.

Variability of Results:

The aim of this book is to aid individuals in enhancing their overall health through informed dietary choices. However, it is acknowledged that individual results can vary significantly. Factors such as genetics, lifestyle, medical history, and program adherence play a crucial role in the effectiveness of the strategies discussed.

Priority of Professional Medical Advice:

In instances where the advice provided in this book conflicts with recommendations given by a reader's doctor or healthcare provider, it is imperative that the individual adhere to the professional guidance of their healthcare provider. The information in this book is not intended to replace or supersede any advice or prescriptions provided by medical professionals.

Medication and Treatment:

Readers are cautioned against making any changes to their medication or treatment plans without first consulting with their healthcare provider. Stopping medication or altering treatment regimens without professional guidance can have serious health consequences.

Liability Limitation:

The author(s) and publisher of "2024 Low Glycemic Index & Load Diabetes Diet" shall not be held liable for any direct, indirect, incidental, consequential, or any other damages that may arise from the use, or misuse, of the information provided. Readers assume full responsibility for any actions taken based on the information contained in this book and agree to use discretion and seek professional advice when necessary.

CONTENTS

THE DIABETES-FRIENDLY CARBS, PROTEINS, FATS AND FIBER COUNTER

THE GI, GL & NET CARB COUNTER

INTRODUCTION

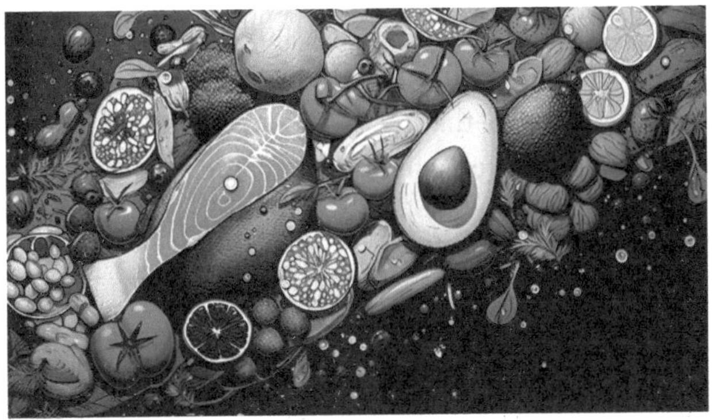

Success in diet management, particularly for diabetes, relies significantly on how you manage carbohydrate intake. Although current Centers for Disease Control and Prevention (CDC) guidelines suggest that about 45-50% of our daily caloric intake should come from carbohydrates, the real challenge in diabetes management transcends these percentages. It involves understanding how different carbohydrates affect blood sugar levels and integrating this knowledge into daily meal planning—a strategy proven to substantially improve glucose control and blood markers.

I developed this awareness over 27 years, not as a patient, but as a pharmacist working closely with those affected by diabetes, witnessing the burdens and poor outcomes of uncontrolled diabetes due to adherence to unfriendly dietary patterns. My extensive experience has allowed me to observe various trajectories of diabetes control, ranging from poor to excellent. Seeing the complexities involved in integrating carbohydrate management into a diabetes diet firsthand has shown me that this aspect of diabetes management is significantly more intricate than in other conditions, such as hypertension or kidney disease. In those conditions, the focus generally lies on restricting specific micronutrients like sodium, phosphorus, potassium, and protein. Unlike these simpler dietary modifications, carbohydrates present unique challenges; their diverse structures and functions affect blood sugar levels in non-uniform ways. This variability highlights the necessity of a sophisticated dietary approach that utilizes tools like the Glycemic Index (GI) and Glycemic Load (GL). These tools help differentiate between foods that stabilize blood sugar levels and those that lead to significant fluctuations, thus supporting more effective diabetes management.

The Low Glycemic Index & Load Diabetes Diet presented in this book offers a comprehensive solution that transcends simple carbohydrate management by embracing the broader principles of healthy eating recommended by the 2020-2025 Dietary Guidelines for Americans. This diet emphasizes the consumption of nutrient-rich, whole, and minimally processed foods, incorporating healthy fats such as polyunsaturated and monounsaturated fats. It addresses the core issues of unhealthy eating patterns by substantially reducing the intake of ultra-processed foods, sugary drinks, advanced glycation end-products (AGEs), and foods high in sodium, saturated, and trans fats. By doing so, the Low GL Diabetes Diet mirrors the essential elements of a balanced and nutritious diet, proving to be an effective, science-backed strategy for managing diabetes and enhancing overall health.

Developed in the early 1980s by Dr. David Jenkins, the Glycemic Index (GI) is a scientifically based scale designed to help individuals with diabetes select foods by indicating how different carbohydrates affect blood sugar levels. However, the initial guidelines provided by the GI were somewhat vague and occasionally led to overconsumption, which proved counterproductive for diabetes management. To address these limitations, Harvard researchers introduced the Glycemic Load (GL) concept in 1997, marking a significant advancement over the GI. This refinement offers a more detailed perspective by taking into account the food's GI value along with the amount consumed. One unit of GL is defined as the effect of consuming one gram of glucose, providing a scale with direct physiological relevance.

With this advancement, the Glycemic Load has become critical in managing diabetes, offering substantial benefits for dietary planning and metabolic health. It classifies foods based on their impact on blood sugar and their carbohydrate content per standard serving size, helping individuals maintain their daily carbohydrate intake within the recommended 45%-50% of total calories. The application of GL principles in meal planning is straightforward, proven, and easily integrated into daily life, enabling better blood glucose control, preventing or halting complications, and improving overall health.

Here, we encapsulate the crucial insights gleaned from current research, emphasizing significant findings:

- **Better Blood Sugar Control**: Eating foods with a low Glycemic Load (GL) helps people with diabetes control their blood sugar levels after meals. This means fewer sudden spikes in blood sugar, making diabetes easier to manage.
- **Less Inflammation**: Foods with a lower GL can reduce inflammation in the body. Inflammation is linked to various health problems and complications, so this is a big plus for overall health.

- **Improved Metabolic Health**: Lowering the GL in your diet can also aid maintain your blood sugar, insulin, and fat levels in a healthier range over time. This supports your body's metabolism both now and in the future.
- **Benefits for Diabetic Conditions**: Some fruits, like grapes, which have low GL, are particularly good for reducing high blood sugar and supporting the health of cells that produce insulin, partly thanks to their natural compounds called polyphenols.
- **Significant Health Improvements**: Diets low in GL have been shown to not only help lower long-term blood sugar levels but also improve cholesterol, body weight, and blood pressure. This kind of diet, when combined with medications, can significantly enhance overall health and diabetes management.

The Practical Low GL Diet Plan for Diabetes Management

Managing diabetes effectively requires careful diet consideration, particularly when choosing foods that are beneficial for stabilizing blood sugar levels. This book is a practical guide to the Low Glycemic Index and Load Diabetes Diet, combining the principles of "GI" and "GL" with the key elements of Mediterranean and balanced diets. This integrated approach enhances glycemic control, prevents complications, and can halt or delay the progression of existing conditions.

Additionally, "The Low GL (Glycemic Load) Diabetes Diet" is not only backed by rigorous scientific research but also enriched by real-life experiences. This diet is the culmination of extensive meta-analyses that draw on successful case studies, avoiding the common pitfalls encountered in diabetes management. It integrates personal stories from individuals who have successfully navigated the complexities of managing diabetes. These anecdotes not only highlight dietary and lifestyle modifications but also delve into the emotional challenges and potential complications that accompany long-term diabetes management.

The effectiveness of the Low GL Diabetes Diet is supported by a vast bibliography, which you can consult at the end of this book. This comprehensive resource compiles the latest scientific findings and expert opinions to provide readers with the most up-to-date information available. The combination of empirical data and personal narratives offers a holistic approach to diabetes management that is both scientifically sound and profoundly personal.

This book not only discusses theoretical concepts but also offers a practical, structured, three-tiered approach to dietary management:

- **Tier One:** Starts with straightforward tools like diabetes-friendly food lists that specify serving sizes.
- **Tier Two:** Introduces a comprehensive macronutrient counter detailing calories, total carbohydrates, fiber, fat, and protein, all adjusted for diabetes-appropriate serving sizes.
- **Tier Three:** Encompasses an extensive glycemic index and glycemic load counter.

By adopting this structured dietary plan, many individuals have witnessed improved glucose control and, in some cases, remission. This approach demonstrates not only the theoretical benefits but also the practical successes of the Low GL Diabetes Diet in managing diabetes and mitigating the risk of complications.

THE LOW GLYCEMIC INDEX & LOAD DIET FOR DIABETES

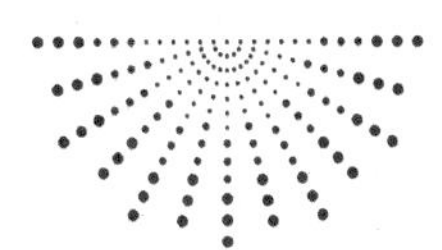

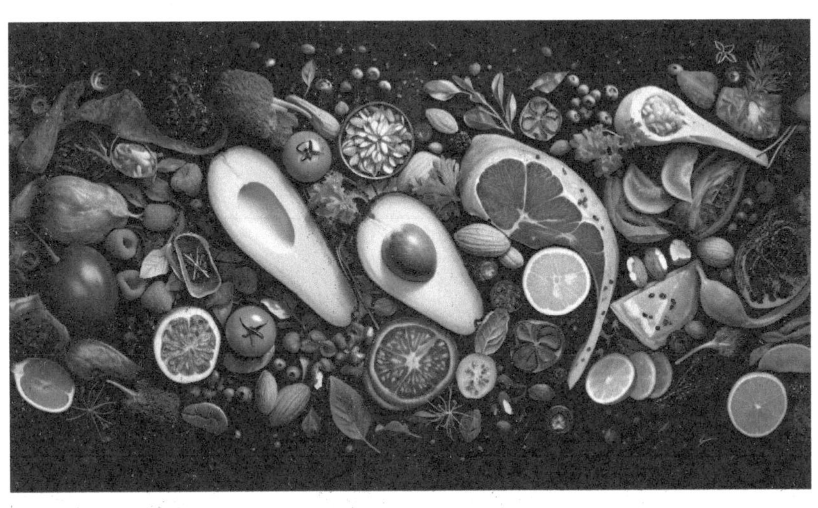

PART I
UNDERSTANDING DIABETES: A COMPREHENSIVE GUIDE

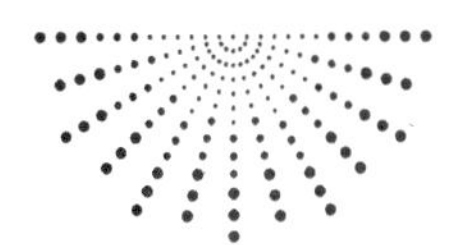

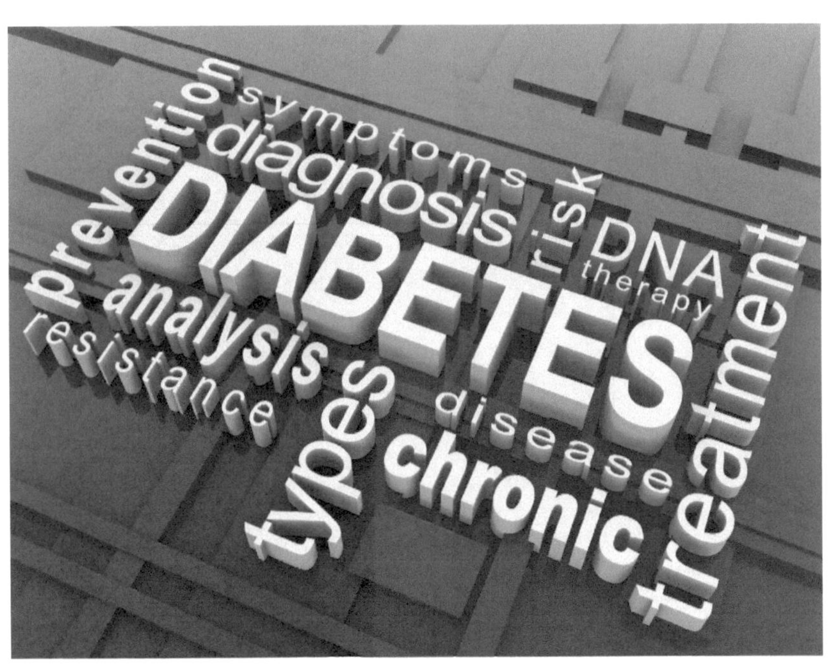

1
DIABETES, INSULIN AND INSULIN RESISTANCE

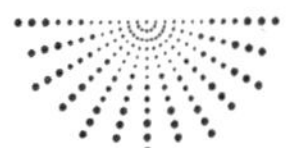

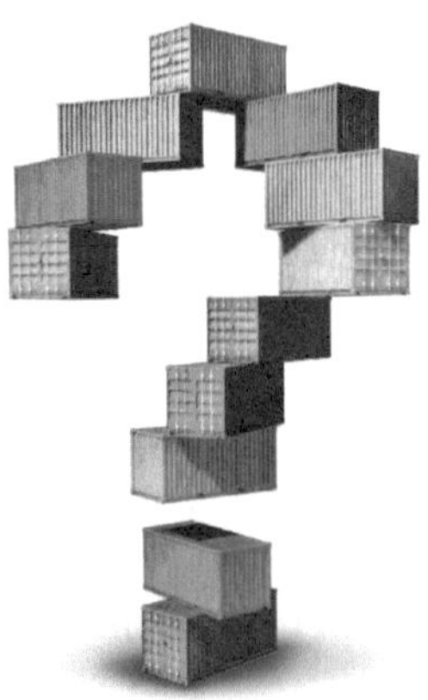

When diagnosed with diabetes or when managing the condition, the term 'insulin' frequently arises. But what exactly is insulin? Is it a medication, a form of treatment, or a natural hormone? And how does it relate to diabetes, including concepts like 'insulin resistance' and 'insulin sensitivity'? This chapter clarifies these questions, providing straightforward explanations and actionable advice.

Understanding Insulin

Insulin is a crucial hormone in human health and one of the most studied hormones due to its vital role in metabolic processes. Produced by the beta cells within the islets of Langerhans in the pancreas, insulin is a protein hormone essential for regulating glucose levels and cell metabolism, and it allows the cellular uptake of glucose for energy production.

Insulin's primary function is to maintain energy balance within the body by managing blood glucose levels. After ingesting food, carbohydrates are broken down into glucose, which enters the bloodstream. Elevated glucose levels trigger the pancreas to release insulin. Insulin aids this glucose in entering the body's cells, where it is used for energy production or stored for future use, thereby helping to regulate the body's metabolic processes.

The infographic below provides a schematic representation of how insulin facilitates the entry of glucose into cells. It outlines four key steps:

1. **Presence of Insulin and Glucose:** Insulin and glucose are available outside the cell, with insulin receptors highlighted on the cell surface.

2. **Insulin Binds to Receptors:** Insulin binds to its receptors, which initiates a signal for glucose channels to activate.

3. **Glucose Entry into the Cell:** The channels open, allowing glucose to enter the cell.

4. **Glucose Utilization:** Glucose inside the cell is used for energy, illustrating effective cellular uptake.

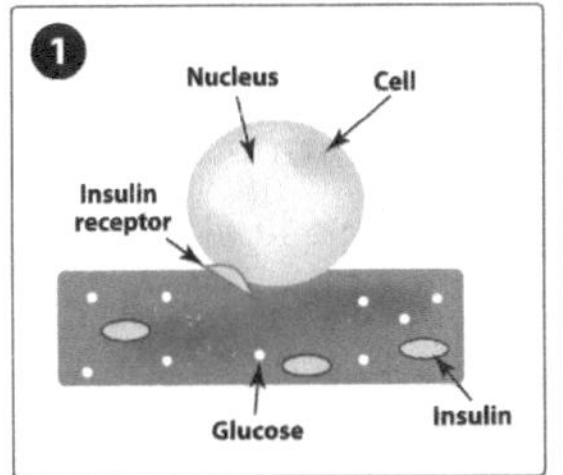

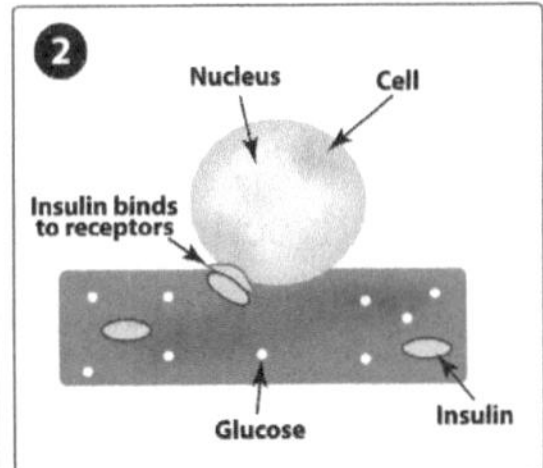

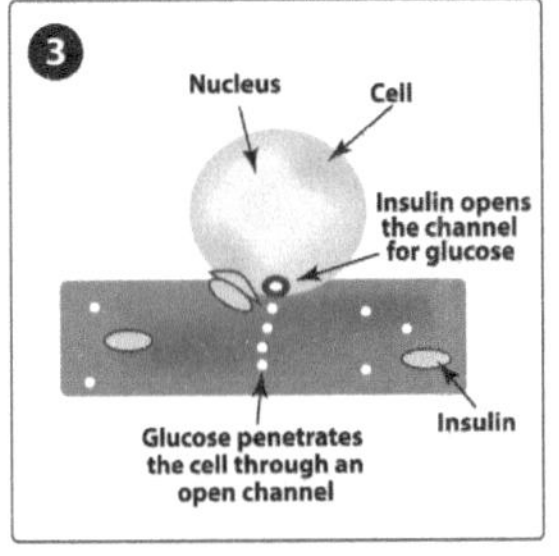

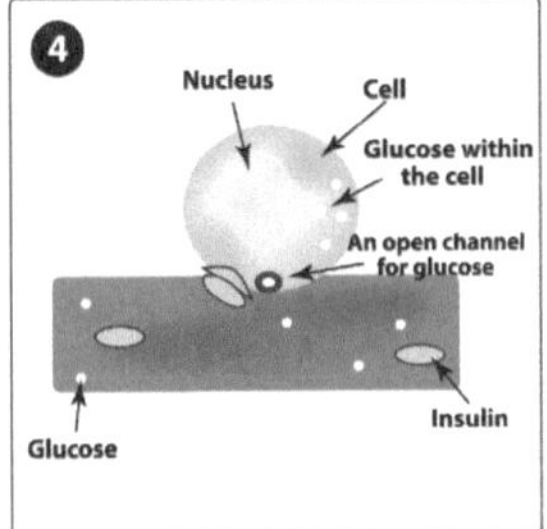

Insulin Action Mechanism Detailed: The infographic "How Does Insulin Work" visually encapsulates the details of insulin's action within the body. Insulin acts like a biological key that unlocks cell membranes, allowing glucose to enter cells from the bloodstream. This process is indispensable for maintaining energy balance and proper cellular function. Insulin binds to an insulin receptor located on the cell membrane, which triggers the glucose channels to transition from a closed to an open state, facilitating glucose's entry into the cell, where it is utilized for energy.

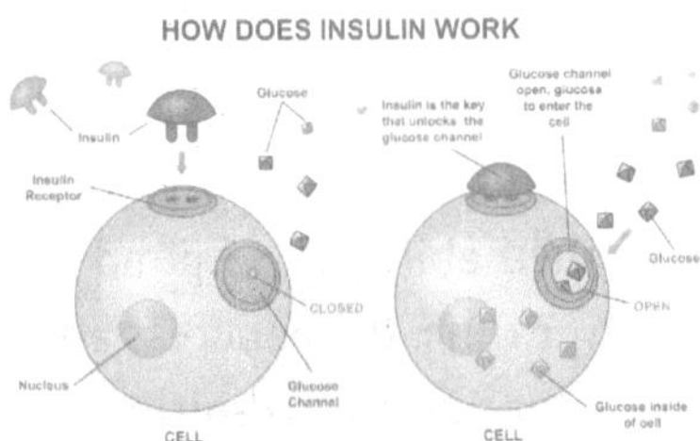

Optimal Blood Sugar Levels: Insulin's pivotal role extends to regulating blood sugar within a healthy range, ideally between 60-100 mg/dL when fasting and under 140 mg/dL after meals. These levels are critical to the body's optimal functioning and help avoid the extremes of hyperglycemia and hypoglycemia. Proper insulin function ensures that glucose is efficiently stored and utilized, maintaining energy balance and metabolic stability. Inadequately controlled blood sugar levels can lead to significant complications, resulting in irreversible damage to organs and tissues.

INSULIN AND DIABETES

Diabetes arises when there is a disruption in insulin's regulatory function. For Type 1 Diabetes (T1D), the body ceases to produce insulin, necessitating lifelong insulin therapy to manage blood glucose levels. This is depicted in the infographic below, showing the mechanism of T1D, where the pancreas produces no insulin, leading to high blood sugar levels as glucose cannot enter the cells.

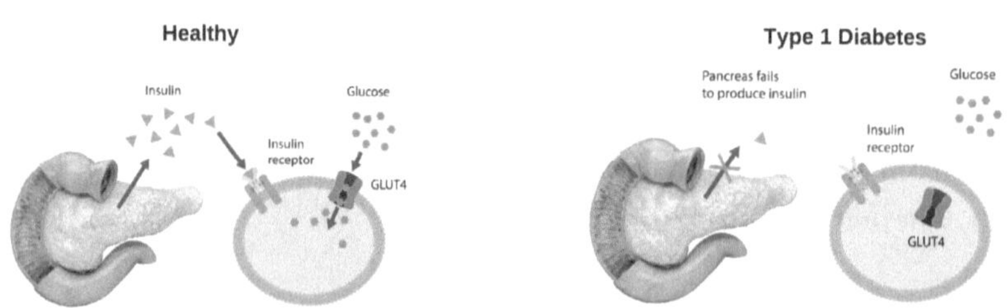

In contrast, Type 2 Diabetes (T2D) typically begins with insulin resistance, where cells lose their ability to respond appropriately to insulin despite its presence. Over time, the pancreas struggles to keep up with the increased demand for insulin, resulting in progressively worse glucose control. Initial management strategies for T2D focus on lifestyle changes, including diet and exercise, to improve insulin sensitivity. As the condition advances, medications that enhance the body's response to insulin may be required, and eventually, some individuals might also need insulin therapy. This progression is visualized in the infographic below, illustrating how the pancreas still produces insulin but at insufficient levels, and the muscle cells do not effectively utilize glucose due to insulin resistance.

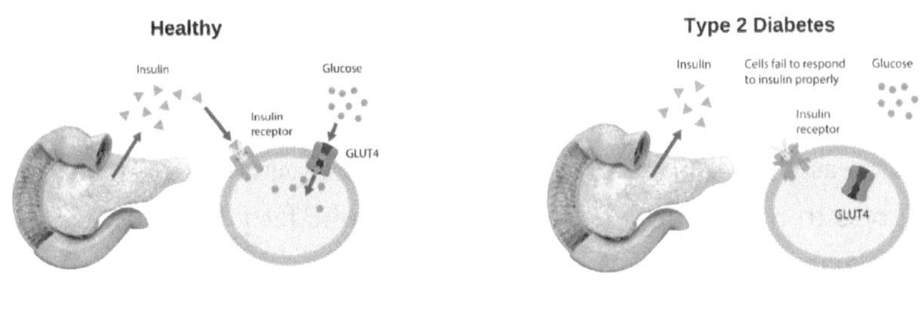

Insulin Resistance and Why You Should Care

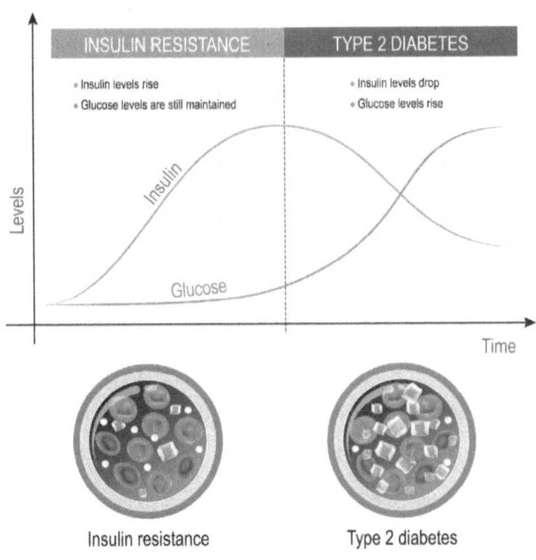

Insulin resistance (IR) is a major global health issue closely linked to obesity and type 2 diabetes (T2D). It disproportionately affects various demographic groups, including certain ethnicities, older individuals, and those from lower socioeconomic backgrounds. Insulin resistance occurs when muscle, fat, and liver cells do not respond adequately to insulin, prompting the pancreas to make more insulin than usual to maintain normal glucose levels. Without dietary changes, insulin resistance can worsen, leading to increased cellular resistance, elevated insulin levels (hyperinsulinemia), and metabolic problems such as high blood sugar, hypertension, dyslipidemia, and an increased likelihood of cardiovascular diseases. These issues may progress to metabolic syndrome, nonalcoholic fatty liver disease, and type 2 diabetes.

Why is Insulin Resistance Critical to Consider if You Have Type 2 Diabetes?

Managing insulin resistance is crucial for controlling type 2 diabetes and preventing its complications. It is vital to keep blood glucose within the target range (before meals: 80 to 130 mg/dL; two hours after meals: below 180 mg/dL). As insulin resistance worsens, the body's demand for insulin increases, which may necessitate medication adjustments. Insulin resistance often coexists with other metabolic disorders, exacerbating diabetes progression and heightening the risk of severe complications such as cardiovascular disease.

Approaches to Managing Insulin Resistance

Addressing insulin resistance through dietary choices, particularly low glycemic load (GL) diets, and lifestyle changes, such as regular exercise and effective weight management, can enhance insulin sensitivity, slow the progression of diabetes, and prevent severe complications, including kidney disease, nerve damage, retinal disorders, heart disease, and stroke. Medications are typically prescribed to help manage blood sugar levels effectively.

The diagnosis of insulin resistance involves various tests, including fasting blood glucose tests, oral glucose tolerance tests (OGTT), HbA1c tests, the Homeostatic Model Assessment of Insulin Resistance (HOMA-IR), and insulin sensitivity tests. Prompt recognition of insulin resistance, coupled with lifestyle modifications and, where necessary, medical interventions, is essential for effective management.

Insulin Resistance in Diabetes: Health Implications

Before writing this section, I pondered its potential impact on clarity for my readers. The previous section offers a comprehensive and concise overview of insulin resistance (IR), often overshadowed by the broader context of diabetes. Typically, once Type 2 Diabetes is diagnosed, the focus shifts to managing blood glucose levels—a practical but not optimal strategy. In contrast, individuals with Type 1 Diabetes rarely consider IR in their management plans, as it is generally temporary in T1D.

Over the years, I've observed that patients with a clear understanding of insulin resistance (IR) manage their diabetes more effectively. Awareness that IR persists beyond the initial diagnosis is crucial for ongoing disease management. These patients adhere to diets designed to improve insulin sensitivity, thereby reducing their reliance on medications, which might otherwise require frequent adjustments or lead to complications. Notably, those who strictly follow a low glycemic index and load diet experience significant improvements in their health outcomes. Achieving this level of success is possible for you as well. Even a basic understanding of these concepts can help you mitigate the progression of IR and prevent the array of negative outcomes associated with it, enhancing overall diabetes management.

Here are some of the main implications of insulin resistance:

1. **Skeletal Muscle Insulin Resistance:** Before Type 2 Diabetes is officially diagnosed, insulin resistance can start affecting the muscles, making it difficult for them to store glucose, which muscles need for energy.

2. **Vascular Endothelial Function:** Insulin resistance can harm the endothelial cells lining the blood vessels, reducing their ability to produce nitric oxide. This can lead to stiffer blood vessels, increasing the risk of heart disease.
3. **Disordered Fat Storage and Mobilization:** Insulin resistance can cause abnormal fat storage and breakdown in the body, setting the stage for diabetes by disturbing the body's metabolic processes.
4. **Body Fat Distribution:** People with more fat around their abdomen tend to have worse insulin resistance, possibly because of different hormone activity in this fat and increased nervous system activity.
5. **First-Phase Insulin Secretion:** A typical problem in Type 2 Diabetes is the loss of early insulin response after eating, which leads to higher blood sugar levels post-meal. Addressing this issue could be a key strategy in diabetes treatment.
6. **Insulin Resistance and Associated Diseases:** Insulin resistance is also linked to other illnesses like polycystic ovary syndrome and certain types of fat distribution disorders, where excess belly fat plays a crucial role in disrupting normal insulin activity.
7. **Insulin Resistance and Atherosclerosis:** Since insulin resistance is associated with a higher risk of large blood vessel diseases, understanding how it leads to these problems is essential for developing effective treatments for patients with insulin resistance.
8. **Beta-arrestin-2 and Insulin Resistance:** Beta-arrestin-2 helps insulin signals work correctly. However, if it's deficient, it can contribute to worsening insulin resistance and diabetes progression. Boosting levels of beta-arrestin-2 might improve insulin sensitivity.

2

UNDERSTANDING TYPE 1 AND TYPE 2 DIFFERENCES

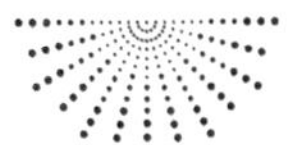

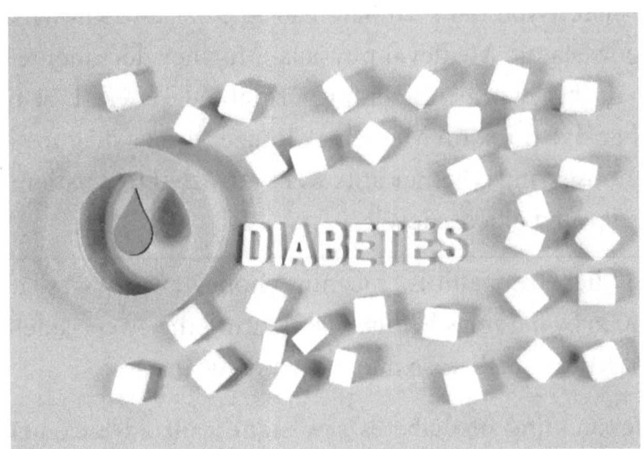

A Brief History of Diabetes

Diabetes mellitus is a common metabolic condition where individuals experience chronic hyperglycemia resulting from defects in insulin secretion, insulin action, or both. Without appropriate treatment, this disorder can escalate into life-threatening complications. Diabetes is primarily classed into two types: Type 1 diabetes (T1D), which is insulin-dependent, and Type 2 diabetes (T2D), which is non-insulin-dependent.

The recognition of diabetes dates back to ancient civilizations, including those of Egypt, Greece, China, and India. These cultures identified three main symptoms—excessive urination (polyuria), sugar in the urine (glycosuria), and intense thirst (polydipsia)—all of which contribute to gradual body wasting, underscoring the disease's catabolic nature.

One of the earliest and most complete descriptions of diabetes was made by Aretaeus of Cappadocia, a physician of the late Hellenistic period in the 2nd century AD. He provided detailed observations of the symptoms and progression of what he called "the melting down of flesh and limbs into urine."

Centuries later, Abu Bakr Muhammad Al-Razi, also known as Rhazes, an eminent Islamic Medieval physician, further documented diabetes mellitus in his works, including "Kitab al-Hawi fi al-tibb" (The Comprehensive Book on Medicine). Rhazes used a diagnostic method involving observing whether ants were attracted to a patient's urine—a sign of elevated glucose levels.

The term "diabetes mellitus," meaning "honey-sweet," was later coined in the 1600s by Thomas Willis, highlighting the sweet-smelling urine characteristic of the disease due to excess sugar.

The understanding of diabetes saw significant advancements in the early 20th century with Frederick Banting and Charles Best's discovery of insulin in 1923. This milestone, which earned them a Nobel Prize, revolutionized the treatment of diabetes, especially Type 1. Subsequently, in 1936, Sir Harold Percival Himsworth differentiated Type 1 from Type 2 diabetes by identifying insulin resistance as a key factor in Type 2 diabetes.

Following the life-saving discovery of insulin, researchers made further refinements and improvements, including the development of longer-acting insulins and insulin analogs to enhance therapeutic outcomes. The development of home blood glucose monitoring in the 1970s gave patients the tools to manage their blood glucose levels actively, significantly improving individual care.

Recent decades have seen the introduction of new medications that improve insulin sensitivity, reduce hepatic glucose production, and enhance glucose excretion, offering more comprehensive management strategies for Type 2 diabetes. These include metformin, sulfonylureas, thiazolidinediones, GLP-1 agonists, and SGLT2 inhibitors.

Technological advances have made a significant impact, particularly with the introduction of continuous glucose monitoring systems and insulin pumps, which automate insulin delivery and significantly ease the daily burden of disease management. Research into the genetic foundations of Type 1 diabetes and the development of immune therapy is paving the way for potential preventive treatments.

Blood Glucose Regulation - Healthy Individuals

Regulating blood glucose is vital for maintaining health and well-being. In individuals with normal pancreatic function, this regulation is finely tuned. After ingesting foods, particularly those abundant in carbohydrates, the digestive system metabolizes them into glucose, which enters the bloodstream. This rise in blood glucose triggers the pancreas to secrete insulin, a hormone that enables glucose to be taken up by cells throughout the body, where it's used as the primary energy source. Any glucose not immediately needed is stored in the liver as glycogen.

Normal Pancreas Functioning:

Upon detecting a rise in blood glucose, the pancreas responds by releasing insulin, which is essential for glucose to enter cells.

Insulin functions as a key, unlocking cells to enable glucose in blood to move into cells for energy utilization or storage.

During periods when you're not eating, such as overnight or between meals, the pancreas releases another hormone called glucagon. Glucagon signals the liver to degrade stored glycogen and release glucose back into the bloodstream, keeping blood sugar levels stable.

The balance between insulin and glucagon release ensures that the body's cells have a steady supply of glucose while preventing levels from becoming too high or too low.

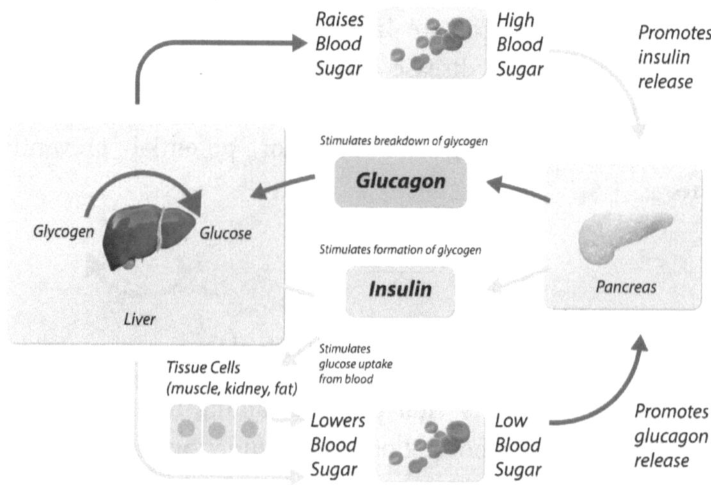

Pancreas Anatomy in Health:

The pancreas is normal in size and shape, with a healthy population of beta cells located within the islets of Langerhans.

These beta cells are responsible for the precise production and regulation of insulin in response to blood glucose levels.

There are no pathological changes or abnormalities present, and the pancreas's alpha cells secrete glucagon as needed.

TYPE 1 DIABETE

UNDERSTANDING TYPE 1 DIABETES

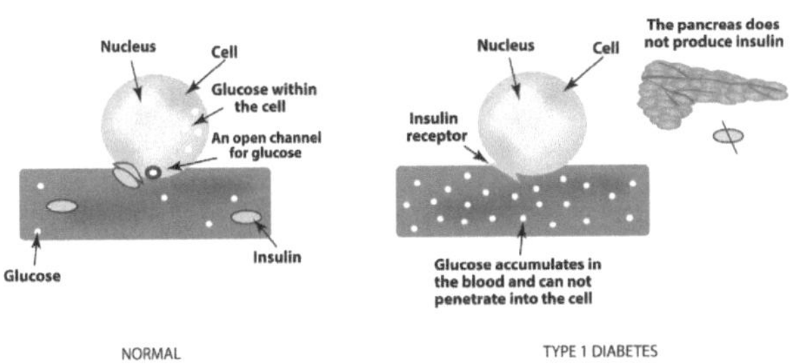

Type 1 diabetes (T1D) is a complex disorder influenced by multiple genetic factors and is classified as an autoimmune disease. In T1D, the immune system attacks the pancreatic beta cells, leading to their progressive destruction and the inability of the pancreas to make insulin. This process is irreversible, causing blood sugar to build up due to the pancreas's reduced capacity to produce this essential hormone. Daily insulin injections and careful dietary management are crucial for survival and minimizing serious health complications. T1D can occur at any age but is most commonly diagnosed in children and young adults. Unlike Type 2 diabetes, T1D is not primarily caused by lifestyle factors, although genetic predisposition and environmental factors, such as certain viral infections, can influence its development.

Type 1 Diabetes Pancreas Functioning:

1. After eating, individuals with T1D experience a rise in blood

glucose due to the absence of insulin secretion following the autoimmune destruction of beta cells.

2. The lack of insulin prevents glucose from entering cells, causing persistent hyperglycemia.
3. The liver, unaware of the high glucose levels due to the absence of insulin, releases more glucose, adding to the already high blood sugar.
4. Energy production is compromised without insulin; external insulin is required for glucose management.
5. People with T1D rely on lifelong insulin therapy as their bodies cannot naturally regulate blood sugar levels.

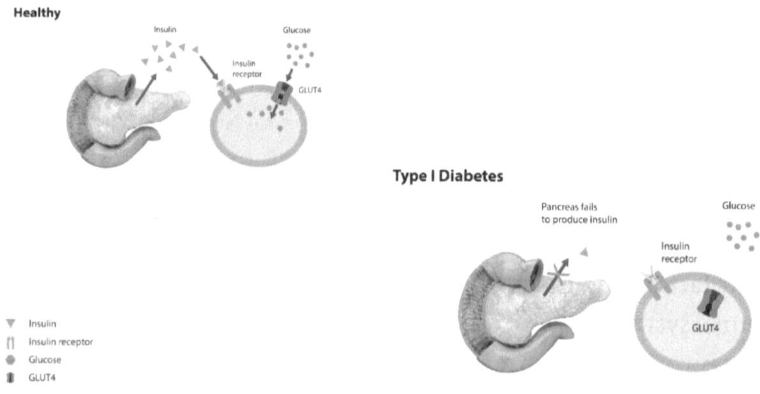

Pancreas Anatomy in Type 1 Diabetes:

- The pancreas may appear smaller due to the significant loss of beta cells.
- Insulitis, or inflammation of the islets, is typically observed, particularly in the early stages, marked by immune cell infiltration and beta-cell destruction.
- The anatomical changes lead to a marked deficiency in insulin production.

Advancements in Treatment:

In 2016, the FDA approved the artificial pancreas, a significant development in T1D management. These devices mimic the function of a healthy pancreas by automatically monitoring blood glucose levels and administering insulin as needed, providing a more stable and responsive treatment method.

Risk Factors for Type 1 Diabetes

Type 1 diabetes (T1D) is influenced by multiple risk factors, some of which are well-documented, while others remain the subject of ongoing research. Key factors known to increase the risk of developing T1D include:

- Family History: The likelihood of developing T1D is higher for individuals with a close relative — such as a parent, sibling, or child — who has the disease.
- Ethnicity: Caucasian individuals in the United States have a higher incidence of T1D compared to African American, Hispanic/Latino, and other ethnic groups.
- Age: T1D is commonly diagnosed in children and adolescents, although it can manifest at any age. The incidence among teens and young adults has been noted to be increasing.
- Viral Infections: Certain viral infections — for example, coxsackievirus B, mumps, and cytomegalovirus — have been implicated in triggering autoimmune response that leads to T1D, potentially by causing disruptions in immune system function.
- Vitamin D Deficiency: Adequate vitamin D levels are essential for immune regulation.

Symptoms of Type 1 Diabetes

The symptoms of T1D often appear abruptly and can quickly become severe. Common symptoms include:

- Frequent Thirst and Urination: Excess sugar in the

bloodstream leads to increased fluid extraction from tissues, causing thirst. Consequently, there is an increase in urine production.

- Intense Hunger: Despite eating, the lack of insulin prevents glucose from entering cells, prompting intense hunger signals.
- Diabetic Ketoacidosis (DKA): Characterized by a distinctive fruity odor on the breath, DKA is a severe condition that results from the body resorting to burning fat for energy due to insufficient glucose entering cells.
- Unexplained Weight Loss: Despite consuming more food to satisfy hunger, weight loss can occur as the body metabolizes muscle and fat as energy sources.
- Blurred Vision: Elevated blood sugar levels can result in the extraction of fluid from the lenses of the eyes, impacting the ability to focus.
- Abdominal Pain: accompanied by feelings of nausea and vomiting, abdominal pain can be a symptom of elevated blood sugar levels.
- Frequent Infections: T1D can weaken the immune system, leading to recurrent infections, particularly in the urinary tract.
- Fatigue: The inability to use glucose for energy can result in persistent tiredness and weakness.

Recognizing these symptoms early is crucial for timely diagnosis and management of T1D to prevent complications and stabilize blood sugar levels.

TYPE 2 DIABETES

UNDERSTANDING TYPE 2 DIABETES

TYPE 2 DIABETES

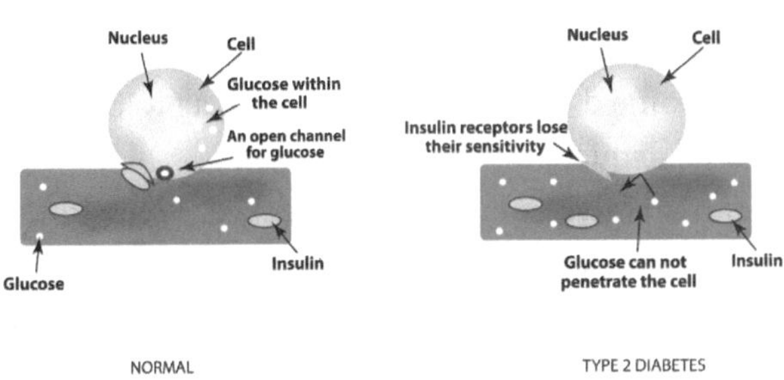

Type 2 Diabetes (or T2DM) is a prevalent metabolic illness resulting from a combination of insulin resistance and pancreatic beta-cell dysfunction. Initially, the pancreas responds to insulin resistance by increasing insulin production. However, over time, this response may become inadequate due to the progressive nature of the disease. Molecular mechanisms that regulate insulin synthesis, release, and action are complex and highly regulated. Any defects in these processes can disrupt the metabolic balance, contributing to the development and progression of T2DM. This form of diabetes accounts for the majority of cases and can occur at any age, though it's most common after forty. In recent times, with the rise in obesity rates and poor dietary choices, T2DM is increasingly affecting younger populations.

Type 2 Diabetes Pancreas Functioning:

In T2DM, the body's cells resist insulin, which hampers glucose absorption and utilization.

1. The pancreas attempts to overcome this resistance by

producing more insulin, but the increased demand may lead to beta-cell fatigue and eventual decline in insulin production.

2. As pancreatic output falters, glucose accumulates in the bloodstream, leading to chronic hyperglycemia.
3. The liver may inappropriately release more glucose into the blood, further exacerbating the condition.
4. Over time, the pancreatic beta cells suffer from overexertion and may become dysfunctional, contributing to the inability to maintain adequate insulin production.
5. Persistent hyperglycemia, if left unchecked, necessitates medical intervention to avoid further complications and to manage blood sugar levels effectively.

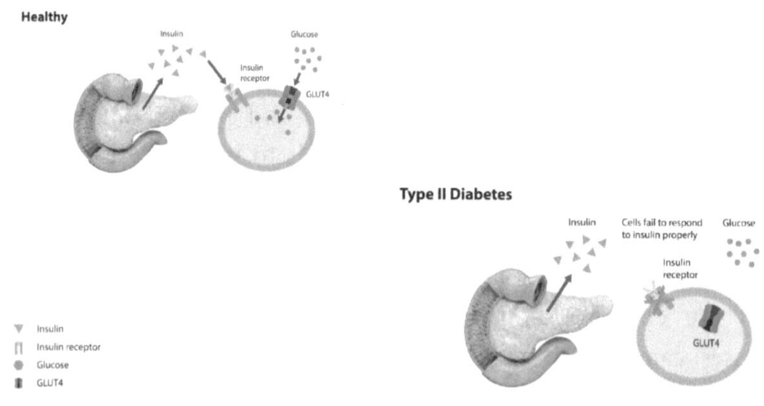

Pancreas Anatomy in Type 2 Diabetes:

• The pancreas in T2DM might vary in size; some individuals may have an enlarged pancreas due to initial beta-cell overactivity in response to insulin resistance.

• Beta cells in the pancreas show signs of dysfunction and may decrease in number, contributing to a reduced capacity for insulin production.

• Amyloid deposition within the islets of Langerhans is a common finding in T2DM, which can disrupt normal insulin secretion and exacerbate the disease.

Risk Factors for Type 2 Diabetes

Type 2 Diabetes (T2D) arises from a combination of genetic, lifestyle, and environmental factors. Key risk factors include:

- Overweight and Obesity: Excess body weight, particularly around the abdomen, is a significant predictor of T2D.
- Family History: Individuals with a family history of T2D are more likely to develop the condition, underscoring a genetic predisposition.
- Ethnic Background: T2D incidence is higher in certain ethnic groups, including African Americans, Hispanics/Latinos, American Indians, and Asian Americans.
- Age: While typically diagnosed in adults over 45, T2D is increasingly occurring in younger individuals, paralleling the rise in obesity rates.
- High Blood Pressure: Hypertension is often associated with an increased risk of T2D and heart and vascular diseases.
- Polycystic Ovary Syndrome (PCOS): Women with PCOS are at greater risk due to the insulin resistance often associated with this condition.
- Vitamin D Deficiency: Adequate vitamin D levels are essential for insulin function and glucose metabolism, with deficiency linked to an increased risk of insulin resistance.

Symptoms of Type 2 Diabetes

The symptoms of T2D often develop slowly and can be subtle, leading to delayed diagnosis. Notable symptoms include:

- Increased Thirst and Urination: Elevated blood sugar levels prompt the kidneys to eliminate surplus glucose through urine, leading to dehydration and increased thirst.

- Weight Loss: Despite consuming more food to compensate for energy loss, weight loss can still occur as the body utilises fat reserves as an alternative energy source.
- Fatigue: Insufficient glucose entering the cells for energy leads to persistent fatigue.
- Blurred Vision: Temporary vision changes can result from fluid shifting into and out of the eye due to high blood sugar levels.
- Slow Healing: High glucose levels impair the body's healing process, leading to slow wound healing.
- Recurrent Infections: T2D affects the immune system, increasing susceptibility to frequent infections.
- Acanthosis Nigricans: Darkened skin patches, often in the neck, armpits, or groin, can indicate insulin resistance.

These symptoms and risk factors underscore the importance of early detection and proactive management of T2D to prevent complications and maintain health.

3
DIABETES COMPLICATIONS AND RISKS

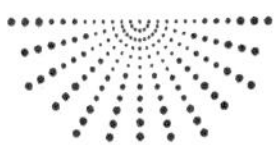

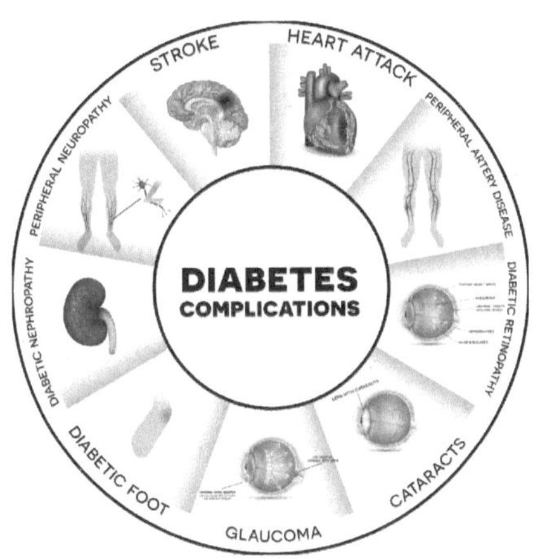

Why We Emphasize the Importance of Understanding Complications?

The rationale behind dedicating an entire chapter to complications, rather than merely listing them, is grounded in the severe and potentially life-altering stakes involved. Diabetes complications can be devastating, significantly affecting quality of life and posing severe health risks. Awareness of these complications alone is insufficient;

it's equally crucial to understand the controllable risk factors to mitigate their impact. This approach goes beyond the basics of diabetes risk factors, delving into the risk factors for complications themselves —an aspect often overlooked in discussions about diabetes.

From Manageable Condition to Severe Threat

When managed with diligent care, including diet, lifestyle modifications, and medication, diabetes can be a manageable condition, imposing minimal restrictions on life. However, absent vigilant management, diabetes morphs into a menacing presence capable of inflicting extensive damage across the body. The spectrum of microvascular to macrovascular complications, including neuropathy, nephropathy, retinopathy, cardiovascular diseases, stroke, and peripheral vascular disease, paints a vivid picture of potential scary outcomes. The progression to peripheral vascular disease, with its dire consequences of non-healing wounds, gangrene, and possible amputation, starkly illustrates the severity of neglect.

Grasping the Gravity of Complications

Recognizing the severe nature of these complications is essential for treating diabetes management as a non-negotiable priority. Understanding the risk factors for diabetes-related complications empowers you to act decisively against them. This real-world observation, drawn from countless patient experiences, underscores the stark reality that neglecting rigorous diabetes management, including risk factor mitigation, dietary intervention, and lifestyle modifications, can lead to severe complications. Many find themselves trapped in a cycle of progressively increasing medication adjustments, unaware of the critical need to halt the disease's progression early on. As diabetes progresses, the rate at which complications intensify can escalate rapidly, underscoring the necessity for early and assertive management strategies. The relationship between diabetes and diabetic kidney disease (DKD) vividly illustrates this point, serving as a sobering reminder of the importance of prevention and the imperative for intensified efforts if complications arise.

Transitioning to the Broader Implications of Diabetes Complications

It's within this context that we recognize diabetes as a leading cause of significant health complications and mortality in the United States, with a profound impact on healthcare costs. The severity of diabetes complications, which can be both devastating and life-threatening, often stems from chronic high blood sugar compounded by other conditions such as hypertension. Although the initial mechanisms—where excess glucose in the bloodstream inflicts damage on the body's vessels and organs—may seem straightforward, the progression of these complications is inherently complex and multifaceted.

Taking chronic kidney disease (CKD) as a prime example, we see a condition deeply feared in the context of diabetes. CKD arises when elevated glucose levels strain the kidneys' filtering capacity to its limits, initiating a series of damages to the nephrons, the kidneys' microscopic filtering units. Diabetic kidney disease (DKD), as identified by Mogensen in the 1980s, starts with microalbuminuria and, without intervention, can advance to macroalbuminuria, signaling a deterioration in kidney function.

As diabetes progresses, its interaction with CKD becomes increasingly complex. Beyond the early stages, where the direct impact of high glucose levels harms the kidneys, the aggravation of CKD further complicates diabetes, weaving a dense web of mutual exacerbation. This intricate and non-linear progression highlights the critical importance of proactive diabetes management. It's not just about managing diabetes in isolation but understanding and addressing the interplay with conditions like CKD to prevent a cascade of complications, emphasizing the necessity of a comprehensive approach to care that considers the wide-reaching implications of this chronic disease.

Exploring the Complexities of Diabetes and Its Complications

Understanding the intricate relationship between diabetes and its complications is essential. Both Type 2 Diabetes (T2D) and Type 1

Diabetes (T1D) present unique challenges but share many complications that can have profound effects on the body's organs and systems. By delving deeper into the specific complications associated with T2D and T1D, we aim to highlight the extensive range of issues that can arise, underlining the critical need for comprehensive management strategies.

Common Complications Across Diabetes Types:

- **Cardiovascular Disease:** Diabetes exacerbates the risk of cardiovascular issues by promoting atherosclerosis, where chronic high blood sugar levels cause inflammation and injury to blood vessels. This leads to plaque buildup, increasing the risk of heart disease, heart attacks, and strokes.
- **Neuropathy:** Long-term high blood sugar can damage nerves, causing neuropathy. Symptoms include numbness, tingling, pain, and weakness, primarily affecting the extremities. This can drastically reduce quality of life, making everyday activities challenging.
- **Nephropathy:** The kidneys' vulnerability to diabetes can lead to diabetic nephropathy, progressing to chronic kidney disease (CKD). This complication may require dialysis or a kidney transplant, highlighting the importance of early detection and management.
- **Ophthalmic Complications:** Diabetes can damage the retina's blood vessels, causing diabetic retinopathy. Untreated, it can develop into severe vision impairment or blindness, underscoring the importance of regular eye exams.
- **Peripheral Vascular Disease:** Impaired blood flow, especially to the limbs, can result from diabetes, increasing the risk of ulcers, non-healing wounds, and potentially leading to amputation in severe cases of infection or gangrene.
- **Dental Health Issues:** Diabetes is linked to deteriorating oral health, including gum diseases, cavities, and increased plaque

formation. Regular dental care is vital to prevent serious dental issues.

- **Immune System Weakening:** Diabetes can compromise the immune system, increasing susceptibility to infections and slowing wound healing, necessitating vigilant care and prevention strategies.
- **Mental Health Concerns:** Managing diabetes's chronic nature can be mentally taxing, potentially leading to anxiety and depression. This underscores the importance of addressing the psychological aspects of diabetes care and ensuring patients receive support for their mental and physical health.

T1D-Specific Challenges:

While T1D and T2D share many complications, the autoimmune nature and typically earlier onset of T1D require additional vigilance. Individuals with T1D may face a higher or more rapid progression of these complications, making early intervention and continuous management paramount. The distinct challenges of T1D, including its unpredictable blood sugar variations and the constant need for insulin management, demand a tailored approach to complication prevention and treatment.

Expanding the Scope of Diabetes Management:

Expanding our understanding of the spectrum of complications associated with diabetes can help us better appreciate the necessity for a comprehensive approach to diabetes care. This includes regular monitoring for early signs of complications, personalized treatment plans that address both T1D and T2D's unique challenges, and comprehensive support that encompasses the physical, dental, and mental health of individuals with diabetes. Recognizing the broad and deep impact of diabetes complications is the first step toward mitigating their effects and improving the lives of those affected by this chronic condition.

Understanding and Managing Risk Factors for Diabetes-Related Complications

In the opening of this chapter, I stressed the importance of not only being aware of the complications associated with diabetes but also understanding and managing the controllable risk factors that can significantly reduce their severity. This proactive approach is not limited to general diabetes risk factors but also encompasses those linked explicitly to complications, emphasizing the vital role of individual actions in improving health outcomes.

The CDC's National Diabetes Statistics Report is an invaluable resource that provides a detailed overview of the risk factors for complications in U.S. adults diagnosed with diabetes. This information, along with other critical diabetes statistics, is accessible on the CDC website via the CDC National Diabetes Statistics Report. (link: https://www.cdc.gov/diabetes/data/statistics-report/index.html)

Reduce Stressors
Increase Activity Level
Reduce Salt Consumption
Reduce Blood Pressure
Prevention of Diabetes Complications
Undergo Health Check up Regularly
Lower Weight
Limit Sugar Intake
Eat More Fiber

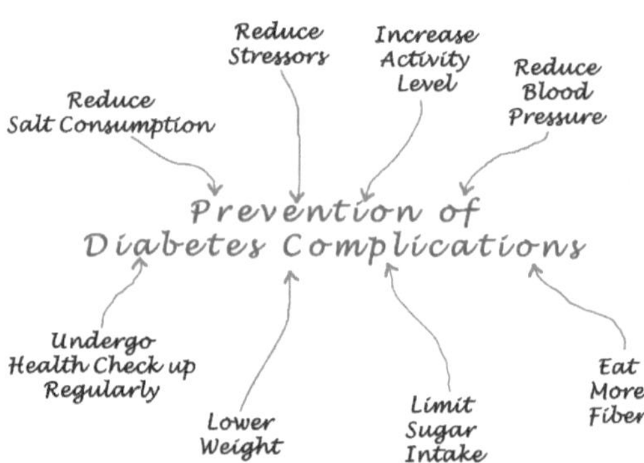

Key Controllable and Modifiable Risk Factors (2017–2020 Data):

- **Smoking Habits:**

- 22.1% of adults with diabetes use tobacco, as identified through self-reports or serum cotinine levels.
- 14.6% are current cigarette smokers.
- 36.0% are former smokers who have smoked at least 100 cigarettes in their lifetime.

- **Body Weight:**

A concerning 89.8% are categorized as overweight or obese (BMI ≥ 25 kg/m^2):

- 26.9% are overweight (BMI 25.0 to 29.9 kg/m^2).
- 47.1% are obese (BMI 30.0 to 39.9 kg/m^2).
- 15.7% are extremely obese (BMI ≥ 40.0 kg/m^2).

- **Physical Inactivity:**

- 31.9% engage in less than 10 minutes per week of moderate to vigorous physical activity, indicating a significant lack of exercise.

- **A1C Levels:**

- 47.4% have an A1C level of 7.0% or higher, indicating suboptimal blood sugar control:
- 22.9% with A1C of 7.0% to 7.9%.
- 11.5% with A1C of 8.0% to 9.0%.
- 13.0% with A1C greater than 9.0%.

- **High Blood Pressure:**

- 80.6% have high blood pressure or are on prescription medication for hypertension (systolic ≥ 130 mmHg or diastolic ≥ 80 mmHg).

- 70.8% have more severe hypertension or are on medication for it (systolic ≥ 140 mmHg or diastolic ≥ 90 mmHg).

High Cholesterol:

- 39.5% have elevated non-HDL cholesterol levels (≥ 130 mg/dL), with detailed breakdowns:
- 19.9% between 130 to 159 mg/dL.
- 11.5% between 160 to 189 mg/dL.
- 8.0% of 190 mg/dL or higher.

Non-HDL cholesterol, including all atherogenic lipoproteins such as LDL, VLDL, and lipoprotein(a), is considered a more accurate indicator of cardiovascular disease risk than LDL cholesterol alone.

The significance of these findings is their potential for control and modification. By proactively managing these risk factors, you can substantially reduce their risk of experiencing severe complications.

4
DIABETES TESTS & DIAGNOSIS

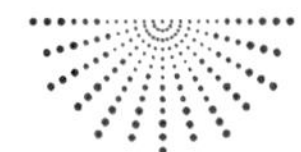

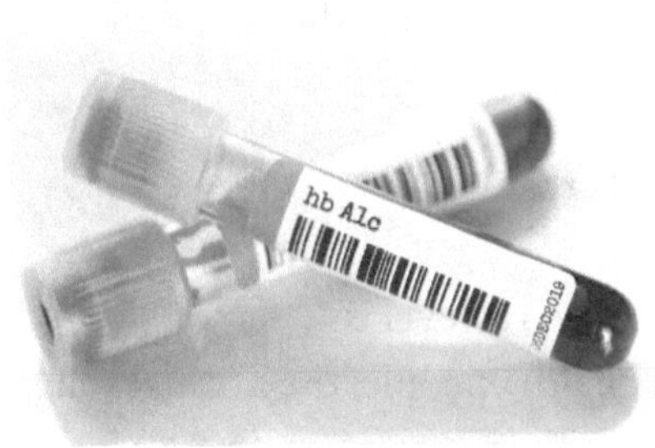

TEST AND DIAGNOSIS

The diagnosis of type 1 and type 2 diabetes typically involves assessing blood sugar levels through various tests, enabling healthcare professionals to make an accurate assessment. Some of the commonly used tests for diagnosing and monitoring type 2 diabetes include:

Fasting Blood Sugar Test:

This test evaluates blood glucose levels following an overnight fast, typically lasting eight hours or more.

Interpreting the FPG results

- An FPG level less than or equal to 99 mg/dL is considered normal.
- An FPG level of 100 **mg/dL (5.6 mmol/L)** to 125 mg/dL **(7 mmol/L)** indicates you have prediabetes and a higher risk of developing diabetes.
- A fasting blood sugar level of 126 mg/dL or higher typically indicates diabetes.

HbA1c Test:

HbA1c Test: This test measures the percentage of hemoglobin in red blood cells coated with glucose, reflecting the average blood sugar level over the past two to three months.

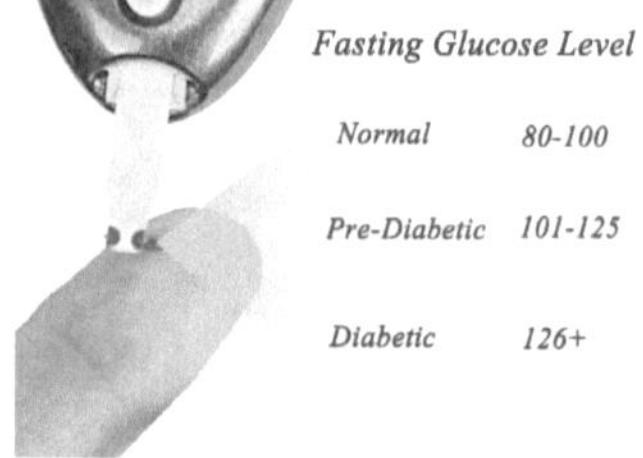

Interpreting the A1C results

- A normal A1C (HbA1c) level is under 5.7%. In healthy people, the normal range for the A1c (HbA1c) level is in the range of 4% to 5.6%
- A level of A1C (HbA1c) in the range of 5.7-6.4% indicates prediabetes and a higher chance of developing diabetes.
- A A1C (HbA1c) level equal to or above 6.5% indicates diabetes.

Oral Glucose Tolerance Test (OGTT):

During the OGTT, the individual consumes a sugary solution, and blood sugar levels are measured two hours later.

Interpreting the OGTT results

- During a 2-hour glucose tolerance test, a blood sugar level of 140 mg/dL or lower is regarded normal.
- A blood sugar level in the range of 140-199 mg/dL indicates you have prediabetes and a higher risk of diabetes.
- A blood sugar level high or equal to 200 mg/dL indicates you have diabetes.

Random Blood Sugar Test:

The random blood sugar RPG test is sometimes used to diagnose diabetes when symptoms are present and when your doctor may need to screen for diabetes without waiting until you have fasted. You may take the RPG blood test at any time. An RPG blood glucose level higher than or equal to 200 mg/dL indicates you have diabetes.

C-Peptide Test: This test measures C-peptide, a byproduct of insulin production, to gauge insulin levels in the body. A C-peptide test helps distinguish between type 1 and type 2 diabetes. Low C-peptide levels may indicate reduced insulin production, suggesting type 1 diabetes. In contrast, elevated or normal C-peptide levels often suggest type 2 diabetes, which is characterized by insulin resistance and relatively preserved insulin secretion.

Upon diagnosis, diabetes management focuses on attaining and sustaining optimal blood sugar levels, preventing complications, and improving overall health and wellness.

5
HYPOGLYCEMIA, A FEARED COMPLICATION OF DIABETES

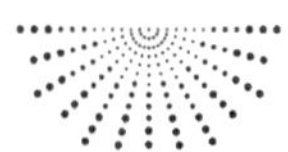

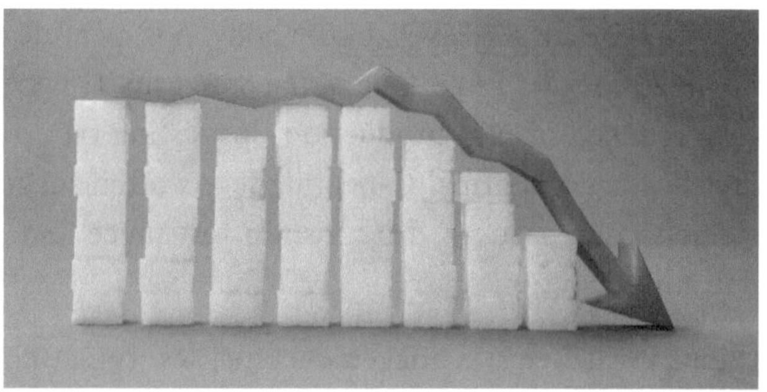

Hypoglycemia, defined as an abnormally low plasma glucose concentration, is a critical issue in the management of diabetes, particularly for individuals relying on insulin therapy, sulfonylureas, or glinides. This condition occurs when plasma glucose levels drop perilously low, posing a significant health risk, especially to individuals with type 1 diabetes, though it can also impact those with type 2 diabetes, albeit at a lower frequency. An extensive international study on insulin-dependent individuals showed that 80% of those with type 1 diabetes and nearly 50% of those with T2D experienced at least one episode of hypoglycemia over a four-week period.

While certain diabetes medications, such as dipeptidyl peptidase-4 inhibitors, metformin, glucagon-like peptide-1 receptor agonists, thiazolidinediones, and sodium-glucose cotransporter-2 inhibitors, generally present a lower risk of hypoglycemia, insulin and insulin secretagogues significantly elevate this risk due to their direct effect on increasing insulin production or release. This inherent risk necessitates meticulous management and monitoring, particularly for patients on complex medication regimens to prevent hypoglycemia.

The American Diabetes Association (ADA) and the European Medicines Agency define hypoglycemia as "any abnormally low plasma glucose concentration that exposes the subject to potential harm," setting a threshold plasma glucose value of <70 mg/dL (<3.9 mmol/L) for this condition.

WHY IS HYPOGLYCEMIA DANGEROUS?

Glucose serves as the brain's primary energy source. Therefore, an acute interruption of glucose supply can result in a rapid cognitive function decline, leading to symptoms ranging from confusion and abnormal behavior to severe outcomes like coma and death. The brain depends on a steady and continuous supply of glucose, as it lacks significant energy reserves. Without prompt treatment, hypoglycemia can impair brain function, causing irreversible harm.

The danger of hypoglycemia lies not only in its immediate impact on cognitive and physical abilities but also in its potential to cause accidents, injuries, and, in severe cases, long-term neurological damage. The risk is compounded during activities requiring concentration and coordination, such as driving.

Moreover, recurrent episodes of hypoglycemia can lead to hypoglycemia unawareness, a condition where the body's normal response to low blood glucose levels becomes blunted. Individuals with hypoglycemia unawareness are at a higher risk of severe hypoglycemia, as they may not recognize or respond to the early warning signs, delaying treatment.

Given these risks, diabetes management strategies that proactively prevent hypoglycemia are essential. This includes careful balancing of medication, diet, and exercise. Utilizing continuous glucose monitoring (CGM) technology and ensuring patients are educated to recognize and respond to the early signs of hypoglycemia are critical steps in mitigating risk.

Prevention of hypoglycemia is preferable to treating it post-occurrence. Individuals with diabetes, especially those at increased risk of hypoglycemia, must be educated about strategies to maintain stable glucose levels. This involves patient and support network education on the early detection of hypoglycemia signs and prompt action to counteract dropping blood sugar levels.

Knowledge of hypoglycemia's symptoms and preventive measures is crucial in diabetes management. This is especially true for patients on medications that carry a risk of hypoglycemia, highlighting the need for a vigilant, informed approach to care.

Diagnosing hypoglycemia entails recognizing its varied symptom onset among individuals, with episodes classified into three levels of severity to guide intervention:

- **Level 1 hypoglycemia** is recognized when plasma glucose levels decrease below 70 mg/dL but stay above 54 mg/dL. This stage signals the need for intervention to prevent progression to more severe symptoms.
- **Level 2 hypoglycemia** is marked by plasma glucose levels dropping below 54 mg/dL, indicating a more significant drop that requires immediate corrective action.
- **Level 3 hypoglycemia** represents a severe episode where mental or physical capabilities are compromised, necessitating help from others for management.

Blood glucose levels fluctuate naturally throughout the day, but readings under 70 mg/dL indicate hypoglycemia. This state calls for quick actions to increase blood glucose levels. In severe cases, hypoglycemia can escalate into a diabetic emergency, making self-treatment impractical and requiring assistance from others. Understanding hypoglycemia's triggers, signs, and symptoms is essential for its effective and timely management.

Symptoms of hypoglycemia typically manifest when blood glucose drops to 70 mg/dL or lower. Although distressing, these symptoms serve as crucial alerts that carbohydrates are needed to correct low blood sugar.

Mild-to-moderate hypoglycemia symptoms include:

- Rapid or irregular heartbeat
- Shaking
- Sweating
- Anxiety or irritability
- Dizziness or lightheadedness
- Hunger

Severe hypoglycemia can lead to:

- Loss of consciousness
- Confusion or disorientation
- Concentration difficulties
- Behavioral changes, such as nervousness or irritability
- Convulsions or seizures
- Coma

Understanding these symptoms is essential for individuals with diabetes to address hypoglycemia and prevent its potentially dangerous consequences promptly.

WHAT LEADS TO LOW BLOOD GLUCOSE IN INDIVIDUALS WITH DIABETES?

Various factors can lead to low blood sugar, including:

- **Over-medication:** Taking too much insulin or medicines that stimulate insulin release.
- **Dietary Mismanagement:** Insufficient carbohydrate consumption, meal delays, or skipping meals, especially when taking insulin or certain drugs.
- **Fasting:** Especially risky while on insulin or glucose-lowering drugs.
- **Excessive Exercise:** Strength training with low carbohydrate intake may cause sudden insulin drops.
- **Weather Conditions:** Hot and humid weather can enhance insulin absorption, raising hypoglycemia risk.
- **Alcohol Consumption:** Especially with heavy drinking and specific medications, the liver may not release enough glycogen to maintain blood sugar levels.

Hypoglycemia Unawareness

This condition occurs when a person does not notice hypoglycemia symptoms. Regular blood sugar checks or continuous glucose monitoring (CGM) devices may be necessary to detect and address low levels promptly.

PREVENTION AND TREATMENT OF HYPOGLYCEMIA FOR DIABETES PATIENTS

Key strategies for diabetes patients to prevent hypoglycemia are:

- **Regular Glucose Checks:** Consistently monitor your glucose levels as per your healthcare provider's recommendations.

- **Consistent Meal Times:** Eat regularly scheduled nutritionally balanced meals.
- **Proper Medication Adherence:** Comply strictly with your prescribed insulin or diabetes medication dosages.
- **Exercise Caution:** Monitor and modify your carbohydrate intake and insulin doses based on physical activity.

TREATMENT FOR HYPOGLYCEMIA

Immediate action is crucial when dealing with hypoglycemia, as it poses a severe risk if untreated.

• **The 15-15 Rule:** For blood sugar levels between 55 and 69 mg/dL, eat 15 to 20 grams of fast-acting carbohydrates and recheck your sugar levels after 15 minutes. Repeat as needed and eat a sustaining meal or snack afterwards.

Options for 15 to 20 grams of fast-acting carbohydrates:

- 3 teaspoons of sugar, honey, or corn syrup
- 3 glucose tablets
- ½ cup (4 oz) of fruit juice or soda
- A slice of bread, a small banana, a medium apple, regular yogurt, or 20 grapes
- ½ cup of cooked couscous or pasta
- 1 cup (8 oz) of milk

Severe Hypoglycemia Management

In cases of severe hypoglycemia, others must act quickly and administer glucagon, available in nasal spray and injection forms, to rapidly increase blood glucose levels. Ensure your family, friends, and coworkers understand how to spot severe hypoglycemia, use glucagon, and know where it is kept.

6

DRUG MANAGEMENT OF DIABETES: INSIGHTS FROM A PHARMACIST'S PERSPECTIVE

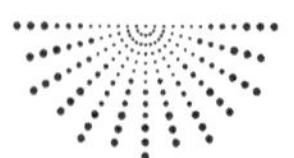

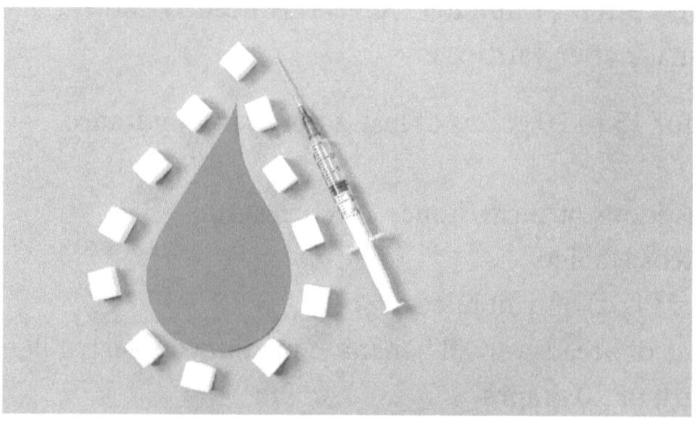

Effective glucose control is central to managing both type 1 and type 2 diabetes, as achieving and maintaining near-normal glycated hemoglobin (HbA1c) levels significantly lowers the risk of macrovascular and microvascular complications. While dietary and lifestyle modifications form the cornerstone of glucose management, most individuals will require pharmacological interventions over time. In type 1 diabetes, the lack of natural insulin production involves the administration of insulin from external sources. Conversely, type 2 diabetes involves progressive loss of beta-cell function, which, if not mitigated through proper diet (e.g., low glycemic index and load diet), leads to worsening metabolic control, necessitating medications to improve insulin sensitivity, augment insulin secretion, or provide insulin in advanced stages.

In the early 1990s, the pharmacological landscape for diabetes treatment was confined mainly to three classes of drugs: insulin, sulfonylureas, and metformin. Since then, the discovery and approval of multiple new drug classes have expanded the pharmacological toolbox available to clinicians. Extensive research has revealed that some of these new classes offer additional benefits beyond glycemic control, such as improvements in cardiovascular health, heart failure management, and kidney disease outcomes.

Today, the array of pharmacological treatments for diabetes encompasses both oral and injectable agents across several classes. These include:

- **Metformin (Biguanides):** The cornerstone of type 2 diabetes treatment, metformin enhances insulin sensitivity, lowers blood glucose levels without causing weight gain, and may even promote weight loss. Its safety profile and effectiveness have made it the first-line treatment, reflecting a deep understanding of its benefits in diabetes management.
- **Sulfonylureas:** This class of drugs stimulates insulin secretion from pancreatic β-cells, effectively lowering blood glucose levels. However, their use is associated with weight gain and an increased risk of hypoglycemia, necessitating careful patient selection and monitoring.
- **Meglitinides:** Similar to sulfonylureas, meglitinides stimulate rapid insulin release but with a shorter action duration. They offer flexibility in dosing but can also cause weight gain and hypoglycemia, making patient education on meal timing crucial to their effectiveness.
- **Insulin Therapy:** For patients with type 1 and advanced type 2 diabetes, insulin is vital. However, its association with

weight gain and the risk of hypoglycemia requires careful monitoring and personalized dosing, highlighting the need for individualized treatment plans.

- **Sodium-Glucose Transport Protein 2 (SGLT2) Inhibitors:** SGLT2 inhibitors reduce blood glucose by promoting its excretion in the urine. They offer the dual benefits of glucose control and weight loss, along with cardiovascular and renal protective effects, marking a significant advancement in diabetes therapy.
- **GLP-1 Receptor Agonists:** GLP-1 receptor agonists lower blood sugar levels while promoting weight loss and offering cardiovascular benefits, reflecting a preference for medications that provide comprehensive health advantages.
- **Oral Glucagon-Like Peptide 1 (GLP-1) Receptor Agonists:** While most GLP-1 receptor agonists are injectable, oral formulations have emerged, offering an alternative route of administration. They improve glycemic control, promote weight loss, and have cardiovascular benefits, aligning with a broader approach to diabetes management that extends beyond glucose regulation.
- **DPP-4 Inhibitors:** With a neutral effect on weight, DPP-4 inhibitors offer an effective, safe alternative to manage type 2 diabetes, emphasizing the necessity for treatments that minimize adverse effects.
- **Thiazolidinediones (TZDs):** Although TZDs enhance insulin sensitivity, they are linked to weight gain, fluid retention, and heart failure risk. Their use underscores the critical need for a careful assessment of benefits versus potential side effects in diabetes therapy.
- **Dopamine Agonists:** This unique class of medication, represented by bromocriptine, has a modest effect on glucose control and is associated with weight neutrality. Its mechanism in diabetes management is distinct, involving circadian rhythm regulation.

OPTIMIZING DIABETES MANAGEMENT: MEDICATION AND LOW GL DIABETES DIET

Effective diabetes management involves more than just medication; it requires a strategic combination of medical treatment and lifestyle changes. Consulting healthcare professionals before adjusting or discontinuing any diabetes medication is essential. At the same time, adopting a low glycemic index and load diet is crucial for enhancing insulin sensitivity and effectively managing blood glucose levels.

Some diabetes medications can cause weight gain and carry significant costs, which can be major concerns. These issues underscore the importance of maintaining an open dialogue with healthcare providers to explore suitable alternatives rather than making independent medication adjustments. Decisions to modify, change, or reduce medications should be made in collaboration with your endocrinologist and pharmacist, who can provide tailored alternatives that align with your health needs and lifestyle preferences.

As we conclude this section, it is essential to highlight the benefits of integrating a low-GL diet with pharmacotherapy. An adequately followed low-GL diet can significantly enhance insulin sensitivity and improve the effectiveness of diabetes medications. However, this may require adjustments to medication dosages under the strict guidance of a specialized healthcare provider. Be vigilant for signs of hypoglycemia, which may indicate improved insulin resistance and a potential need to adjust your medication dosage. These positive changes should be reflected in your A1C and daily glucose monitoring and discussed during your routine visits to the doctor.

7
THE ABCDE OF DIABETES

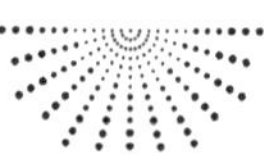

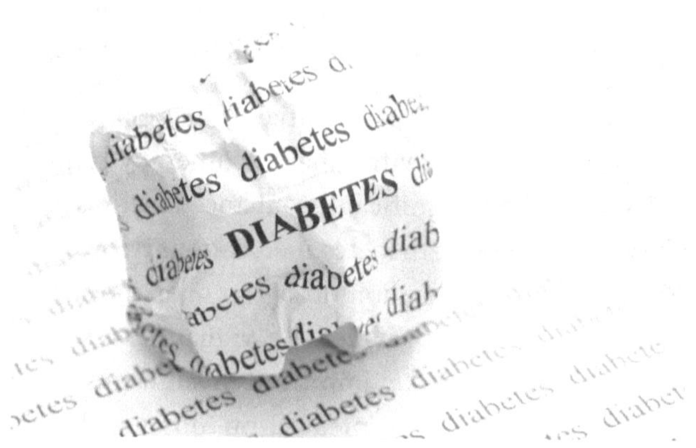

THE ABCDE OF DIABETES MANAGEMENT: A COMPREHENSIVE FRAMEWORK

The ABCDE of diabetes management provide a structured and holistic framework to enhance the effectiveness of diabetes care and improve overall health outcomes. This approach emphasizes the critical aspects of managing diabetes and promotes a comprehensive strategy to boost well-being across various facets of life.

Blood Markers Monitoring and Its Impact

Monitoring key blood markers is pivotal in managing diabetes and preventing complications. Persistent high blood sugar levels can cause a host of issues, including severe hypertension, which affects nearly half of those diagnosed with type 2 diabetes. This condition can constrict blood vessels, adversely affecting vital organs and potentially leading to significant health complications. Moreover, diabetes can drastically alter the lipid profile in the bloodstream, thereby raising the likelihood of cardiovascular diseases. Regular and vigilant monitoring of these markers is crucial to averting such detrimental outcomes.

The Role of Lifestyle Change in Diabetes Management

Managing diabetes effectively extends beyond dietary adjustments; it encompasses a range of targeted lifestyle changes that underpin the overall management strategy and contribute to improved health. This holistic approach highlights the importance of physical activity, proper hydration, and adequate sleep—all essential for better blood sugar control as well as enhanced insulin sensitivity. Regular physical activity and ensuring enough sleep are vital, as they not only help in stabilizing sugar levels but also play a significant role in reducing the risks associated with diabetes-related complications.

STRATEGIC FRAMEWORK: THE ABCDE OF DIABETES MANAGEMENT

A1C (HbA1c) Test: The A1C test is an essential indicator of long-term glucose control, reflecting average blood sugar levels over the two to three last months. For most adults with diabetes, it is advised to keep the A1C level under 7% to minimize the risk of complications like neuropathy, retinopathy, and cardiovascular diseases. However, A1C targets can be individualized based on factors such as age, duration of diabetes, presence of complications, and overall health. For example, stricter targets (below 6.5%) may be set for younger individuals or those without significant heart disease who can achieve such levels without severe hypoglycemia. Conversely, less stringent targets (such as 8% or slightly higher) might be appropriate for older adults, those with complex health issues, or where hypoglycemia risk is a concern. Regular monitoring of A1C levels allows for timely adjustments in treatment plans to meet these personalized health needs.

Blood Pressure Management: Controlling blood pressure is crucial for individuals with diabetes, as hypertension significantly elevates the risk of cardiovascular diseases. Current guidelines generally recommend a target blood pressure of less than 130/80 mm Hg for most people with diabetes. This target can be achieved through lifestyle modifications such as diet, exercise, and pharmacological treatments if necessary. However, targets may be personalized based on individual risk factors and co-existing medical conditions.

Cholesterol Management: Dyslipidemia, characterized by high LDL cholesterol, high triglycerides, and low HDL cholesterol, is prevalent among those with diabetes and raises the risk of cardiovascular complications. Monitoring lipid levels is essential, and treatment should be tailored to individual needs. This often involves dietary adjustments, physical activity, and potentially lipid-lowering medications. Treatment goals typically include lowering LDL cholesterol to less than 100 mg/dL and even lowering it in individuals with additional cardiovascular risk factors. Adjusting these targets might be necessary depending on overall health and specific cardiovascular risk profiles.

Diet and Nutrition: A healthy, balanced, diabetes-focused diet is vital in managing diabetes and preventing its complications. It's essential to balance nutrient intake and include fiber-rich foods while monitoring carbohydrate consumption. Dietary patterns such as the low glycemic load diet, the Mediterranean diet, DASH, and plant-based diets are beneficial for those with diabetes.

Exercise and Physical Activity: Regular exercise is crucial for managing diabetes and enhancing overall health. It improves insulin sensitivity, aids in weight management, and lowers the risk of heart disease. Health guidelines suggest a weekly routine of at least 150 minutes of medium-intensity aerobic activity and activities that build muscle strength.

Personalized Management Considerations:

- **Timely Medications:** Adhering to prescribed diabetes medications is vital for maintaining optimal glucose levels. Consistent medication use is key to achieving target blood sugar levels.
- **Low GI and GL Food Choices:** Opting for foods with a low glycemic impact helps regulate blood sugar levels effectively. A varied diet, including fruits, vegetables, grains, proteins, dairy, and non-dairy alternatives, while limiting unhealthy fats and processed foods, is advisable.
- **Physical Activity:** Steady physical activity is proven to maintain normal glucose levels. It is recommended that you engage in medium-intensity exercise for at least 30 minutes on most days.
- **Regular Glucose Monitoring:** For those with type 1 diabetes and insulin-dependent individuals, monitoring blood sugar levels is crucial. A glucose meter or continuous glucose monitoring (CGM) helps keep glucose levels within the target range.

PART II
KNOWING WHAT'S IN THE FOOD YOU EAT

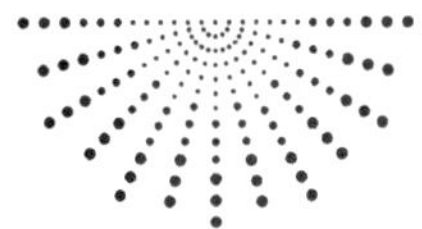

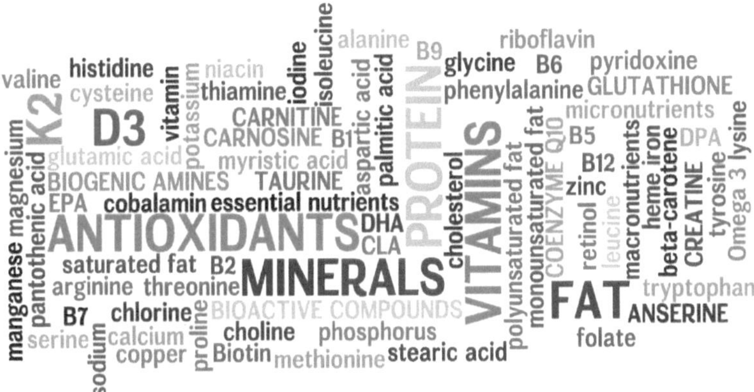

8
CARBOHYDRATE ESSENTIALS: WHAT YOU NEED TO KNOW

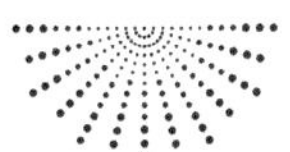

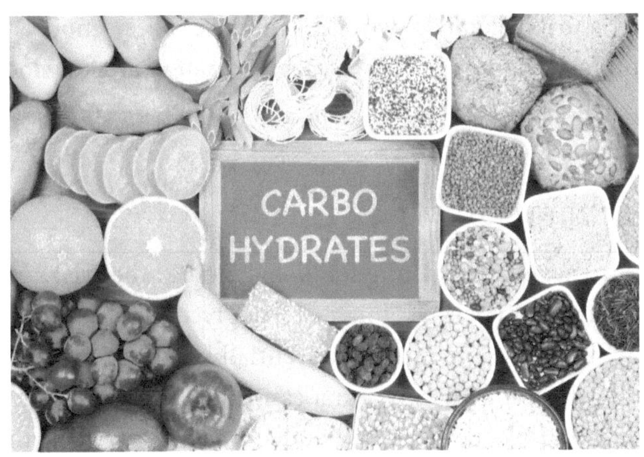

RETHINKING CARBOHYDRATES IN DIABETES MANAGEMENT

Managing diabetes effectively involves more than just restricting carbohydrates; it requires a sophisticated understanding of how various types of carbohydrates impact blood sugar levels. Over the past 25 years, I've noted a common misconception that carbohydrates must be drastically reduced due to their impact on blood sugar.

However, extreme restrictions are neither practical nor beneficial since carbohydrates are essential energy sources that our bodies are designed to utilize.

The popularity of the High Fat, Low Carb (HFLC) diet, which limits carbohydrate intake to as low as 15% of daily calories, aims to manage blood sugar and help in weight loss. Despite its popularity, this diet doesn't consistently deliver results for everyone, often leading to disappointment. Significant reductions in carbohydrate intake usually mean compensating with higher protein and fats, which can lead to health issues such as heightened likelihood of heart disease, gout, and, in individuals with kidney disease, heightened kidney strain due to elevated phosphorus levels.

Our approach to diabetes management has evolved significantly, from using exchange lists in the early 2000s to adopting the Glycemic Index (GI) and Glycemic Load (GL) models. These models reflect a deeper understanding of how carbohydrates affect blood sugar stability.

BALANCING BLOOD SUGAR RISKS

Diabetes management also entails balancing the risks of hypoglycemia and hyperglycemia. Hypoglycemia is particularly dangerous for those on insulin, potentially leading to emergencies. Meanwhile, chronic hyperglycemia can lead to severe complications, such as irreversible damage to vital organs, diabetic ketoacidosis, and coma.

THE IMPORTANCE OF DIETARY FIBER

To mitigate these risks, incorporating a sufficient amount of dietary fiber is essential. I recommend a daily intake of 25 to 30 grams of fiber. Fiber digests slowly, stabilizing blood sugar levels and offering numerous health benefits beyond diabetes management, such as supporting heart health, reducing risk factors for stroke and hypertension, and maintaining gastrointestinal health and a healthy microbiome.

Recent Insights on Dietary Fiber in Diabetes Management

- **Type 2 Diabetes (T2DM) Management**: Research underscores the role of high dietary fiber intake in decreasing T2DM risk, advocating for healthy eating habits for both prevention and management.
- **Gut Health and T2DM**: Dietary fiber has a positive effect on gut bacteria, which is crucial for managing T2DM, boosting immunity, and playing a vital role in overall health.
- **Fiber Supplementation in T2DM (STAR Survey)**: Surveys indicate that physicians recommend fiber supplements for T2DM, noting enhancements in blood sugar levels, weight management, and cholesterol levels. Patients report increased satiety and reduced medication needs.
- **Viscous Soluble Dietary Fiber**: Studies have found that viscous soluble fiber significantly lowers blood sugar and cholesterol levels in T2DM, highlighting its importance in managing glucose and cholesterol.
- **Gestational Diabetes**: Research shows dietary fiber supplements can improve fasting and postprandial glucose levels, HbA1c, and lipid profiles, enhancing pregnancy outcomes.

DETERMINING THE RIGHT AMOUNT OF FIBER

For individuals with diabetes, it is recommended to eat 20 to 35 grams of fiber daily from sources like raw vegetables and unprocessed grains, nearly 14 grams of fiber per 1,000 calories, consistent with guidelines for the general population. Ensuring at least half of your grain intake is from whole grains is crucial. Look for high-fiber carbohydrates (over 5 grams per serving) such as legumes, whole grain breads, cereals, and fruits and vegetables. While aiming for a daily fiber intake of 25 grams or more, it is essential to gradually increase your intake to avoid gastrointestinal issues.

Balancing your carbohydrate intake is crucial, with recommendations suggesting that 45-50% of your total daily calories should come from carbohydrates. This balanced approach emphasizes the importance of focusing on high-quality, fiber-rich carbohydrates for effective diabetes management and metabolic health.

CARBOHYDRATES WITHIN THE LOW GL DIABETES DIET

Building on the foundational insights from the previous section, which emphasized carbohydrate management in diabetes and the essential role of fiber, we now delve into a more detailed exploration of how the glycemic impact of foods can refine our understanding and management of carbohydrates. This section addresses a common query among individuals with diabetes: "What can I eat to maintain my blood sugar levels within the therapeutic target?"

Unlike the broad categorization of carbohydrates and the role of fiber, this segment introduces how carbohydrate-containing foods elicit varying postprandial blood sugar responses. These responses are integral to developing the Glycemic Index (GI), which categorizes foods based on their impact on blood glucose levels. Further, by considering the quantity of carbohydrates consumed, we can determine a food's Glycemic Load (GL), providing insight into its physiological effect on blood sugar.

This advanced understanding is vital for informed dietary choices, especially when evaluating the direct postprandial effects of different foods. While the fiber content and the classification of carbohydrates as simple versus complex offer a preliminary guide, the GI and GL values furnish a more nuanced gauge for making dietary decisions with a comprehensive understanding of a food's glycemic impact.

CARBOHYDRATE CLASSIFICATION: SIMPLE VS. COMPLEX

Carbohydrates are generally divided based on their molecular structure into:

- **Complex Carbohydrates:** Characterized by long, intricate chains of sugar molecules, complex carbohydrates are found in unprocessed foods such as vegetables, fruits, legumes, and whole grains. Their rich fiber content and structural complexity result in slower digestion rates, aiding in stabilizing blood sugar levels.
- **Simple Carbohydrates:** These are rapidly metabolized and absorbed, resulting in quick spikes in blood glucose levels. Predominantly found in processed foods, refined sugars, and snacks, the frequent consumption of simple carbohydrates is tied with health risks such as metabolic syndrome, Type 2 Diabetes Mellitus (T2DM), and obesity.

Carbohydrates are further divided into three main types, each with distinct characteristics and impacts on blood sugar regulation:

- **Sugars:** These simple carbohydrates are made up of short-chain molecules, including fructose (found in fruits), glucose (a fundamental sugar unit), sucrose (table sugar), and galactose (found in milk). Sugars are rapidly metabolized by the body, causing abrupt spikes in blood sugar levels.
- **Starches:** These are complex carbohydrates consisting of long chains of glucose molecules. They break down into glucose during digestion, providing a steadier energy release than sugars. Common sources include potatoes, corn, and whole grains.
- **Fibers:** Unlike sugars and starches, fibers are carbohydrates that the body cannot digest. They are crucial for maintaining digestive health and significantly affect blood sugar control. Fibers are classified as soluble (which dissolve in water and

slow digestion) or insoluble (which promote bowel health and regularity).

NAVIGATING CARBOHYDRATES IN A DIABETES DIET

Standard advice upon a diabetes diagnosis often includes prioritizing complex carbohydrates and minimizing simple carbohydrates and added sugars. While this guidance has merit, it can oversimplify the complexity of simple carbohydrates. For example, fruits contain simple sugars like fructose, sucrose, and glucose, but they also offer vital vitamins and nutrients, making them essential for a balanced diet. Similarly, dairy products provide simple carbs like galactose and natural products like honey contain fructose and glucose. Eliminating these foods from your diet isn't necessary.

Adopting a more refined approach is critical. Not all simple carbohydrates impact health equally. Those found in whole fruits, for instance, are beneficial due to their nutrient density and fiber content, which can moderate their effect on blood sugar levels. In contrast, simple carbs found in processed foods or sugary drinks can negatively impact blood sugar management and overall health.

The distinction between eating a whole fruit and consuming a candy bar—or even a cup of fruit juice—is profound despite potential similarities in sugar content. Whole fruits deliver nutritional value, fiber, and other beneficial compounds, making them healthier than processed sweets or sugary drinks.

Instead of avoiding all simple carbohydrates, it is more effective to choose selectively. Natural sources like fruits and dairy are usually better choices, while processed foods and drinks high in added sugars should be consumed sparingly. This careful selection fosters informed dietary decisions, crucial for effective diabetes management and enhancing overall health.

The Glycemic Index and Glycemic Load

The Glycemic Index (GI) and Glycemic Load (GL) offer a sophisticated, evidence-based framework for meal planning that enhances diabetes management. In the following chapters, we'll explore how to effectively apply GI and GL values to differentiate between beneficial or detrimental foods for diabetes, alongside recommendations for serving sizes and ensuring carbohydrate portions remain around 15 grams. This guidance is designed to illuminate the relationship between carbohydrate consumption and the regulation of crucial hormones, including insulin, leptin, ghrelin, cortisol, and peptide YY —each playing a significant role in managing diabetes.

Furthermore, "diabetes macronutrient distribution" will be explored, empowering you to tailor your diet to meet your health objectives. Despite the challenges posed by diabetes and its potential complications, adopting the correct dietary strategy can lead to successful management of the condition. The focus of this book, the GL Diabetes Diet, equips you with the essential tools and knowledge to live without the constant concern of escalating diabetes issues or complications. This dietary approach will enable you to take charge of your health, paving the way for effective management and a flourishing life despite diabetes.

9
PROTEIN — THE BUILDING BLOCKS OF LIFE

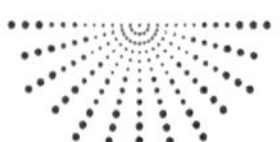

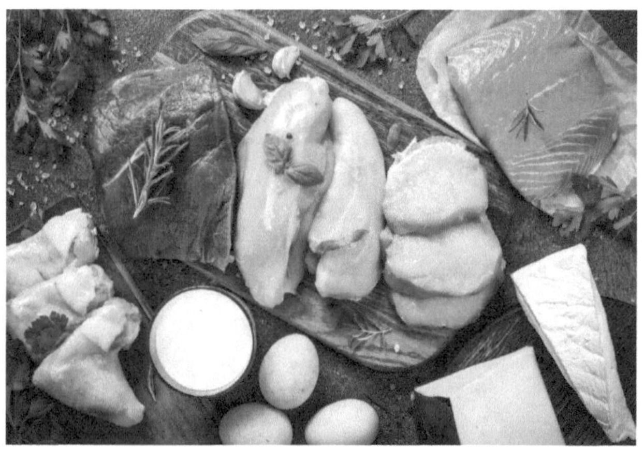

PROTEINS: ESSENTIAL MACRONUTRIENTS

Proteins, alongside carbohydrates and fats, are foundational elements in our diet and vital for maintaining health. They provide the body with amino acids and small peptides, critical for constructing cellular structures and synthesizing essential metabolites, including purines, pyrimidines, and neurotransmitters

Unlike other macronutrients, proteins are unique in their role within the body. They make up about three-fourths of the dry matter in most human tissues, except for bone and fat. These large molecules are not just present, but they are crucial for virtually all vital functions within the body. They serve as catalysts for chemical reactions, regulate gene expression, and are integral to the structure of cells and muscles.

Proteins: Structural and Functional Roles

Within the body, they serve both structural and functional roles. As structural components, proteins are crucial in building and maintaining the physical framework of the body, forming an integral part of every cell, tissue, and organ, including muscles, bones, skin, and hair. They provide the necessary structure that supports the body's overall architecture and physical functionality.

Proteins, with their multifaceted roles, are the unsung heroes of our bodies. They regulate the immune system, ensuring our bodies can effectively respond to pathogens. They facilitate neurotransmission, acting as enzymes, hormones, and receptors that enable cell communication, supporting nerve function and signaling across the nervous system. This dual capacity of proteins to act both as building blocks and as active biological molecules underscores their indispensable nature in maintaining health and supporting essential bodily operations.

The critical role of amino acids

Individual amino acids (AA), the building blocks of proteins, are multifunctional. They act as precursors for hormones and neurotransmitters, vital for communication within the body and overall physiological regulation. For example, the AA tryptophan is a precursor for the neurotransmitter serotonin, which plays a role in mood regulation and sleep.

Proteins are indispensable in the synthesis and repair of tissues, influencing everything from muscle growth to wound healing. Their role in enzyme production is equally important, as enzymes speed up all metabolic processes from digestion to DNA replication. Additionally, proteins contribute to the body's defensive mechanisms by forming antibodies that are crucial to immune response.

This broad range of functions highlights the fundamental importance of proteins in maintaining health and supporting essential bodily operations.

The 9 Essential Amino Acids

From a nutritional perspective, our diets require not directly proteins themselves but rather the nine essential amino acids they provide. These amino acids—histidine, isoleucine, leucine, lysine, methionine, phenylalanine, threonine, tryptophan, and valine—are critical for human health and cannot be synthesized by the body. They must be obtained from dietary sources. A sufficient intake of these amino acids is vital for the production of non-essential amino acids and supports numerous bodily functions, including tissue repair, immune response, and hormone synthesis.

These essential amino acids, which the body cannot synthesize, are found in various animal-based and plant-based foods. This ensures that both omnivores and vegetarians can meet their protein requirements, provided their diet is well-planned. For example, meats, dairy products, and eggs are high-quality protein foods that provide all nine essential amino acids in sufficient amounts. Plant-based foods such as nuts, beans and lentils also provide these amino acids but may need to be consumed complementary to achieve a complete amino acid profile.

THE IMPORTANCE OF PROTEIN IN THE DIET

Unlike fats and carbohydrates, which the body stores as lipid droplets in adipose tissue and glycogen in muscle and liver tissues, proteins lack a specialized storage form. This underscores the importance of regular protein consumption to ensure that the body functions properly. This is especially important during growth, recovery from injury, or when physical activity increases. Additionally, proteins regulate critical physiological processes, such as hormone activity, enzymatic reactions, and immune responses.

Proteins, with their higher thermogenic effect than fats and carbohydrates, play a significant role in metabolic regulation and body composition. They assist in regulating energy expenditure and metabolic rate, contributing to weight management. Moreover, proteins enhance satiety and reduce the desire to consume excess calories, aiding in establishing sustainable eating patterns and effective weight management. This multifaceted role emphasizes their indispensable place in a balanced diabetes diet and the importance of maintaining sufficient protein levels in daily nutrition to support the body's diverse functions.

Protein Intake Guidelines

The RDA for protein, often misunderstood, represents the minimum amount of protein needed to achieve the basic minimal nutritional needs of most healthy individuals, ensuring nitrogen balance in the body. This intake level is crucial to avoid the loss of lean body mass and prevent deficiencies. The RDA, established at 0.8 grams of protein per kilogram of body weight for adults, is meant to avert deficiency rather than indicating the optimum protein intake for improving health and facilitating muscle growth.

Optimal Protein Intake Across Different Groups

The impact of dietary protein on health, particularly for those managing diabetes, obesity, and heart disease, has been extensively studied. Adjusting protein intake based on individual health status, including weight and kidney function, is essential for maximizing health benefits:

- **Normal Weight Individuals with No Chronic Kidney Disease (CKD)**

The Recommended Dietary Allowance (RDA) for protein, set at 0.8 grams per kilogram of body weight per day for adults of average weight who do not have chronic kidney disease (CKD), is designed as a minimum guideline to prevent nutritional deficiency. This intake level is generally considered sufficient to maintain nitrogen balance and prevent muscle loss in most adults. However, emerging research suggests this "minimal" amount is not optimal, especially for those in specific life stages or with increased physical activity levels. For example, higher protein intakes may benefit older adults by supporting muscle mass and strength or athletes aiming to optimize performance and recovery. Therefore, while the RDA serves as a baseline to prevent deficiency, individual needs may vary, and some adults might require more protein to meet their specific health and activity demands. Thus, for those who are physically active, are age 50+, or are seeking muscle growth, protein intake may need to increase to 1.2-2.0 grams per kilogram of body weight per day. This variability in protein needs is crucial to understand, as it underscores the importance of tailoring protein intake to meet specific health and activity demands.

- **Individuals with Overweight or Obesity and Normal Kidney Function**

For individuals who are overweight or obese with normal kidney function, it is suggested to consume protein at levels that might be higher than the RDA for weight management and diabetes control. Intake levels can range from 1.2 to 2.0 grams per kilogram of body weight per day, making up about 20-30% of total caloric intake. This higher protein intake can help with weight loss by promoting satiety and boosting metabolic rate, while also favorably affecting blood pressure, cholesterol levels, and inflammation markers.

- **Individuals with Diabetes and Early-Stage Chronic Kidney Disease (CKD)**

For those diagnosed with diabetes and early-stage CKD, it's crucial to manage protein intake to slow the progression of kidney disease. The American Diabetes Association recommends limiting protein intake to 0.8–1.0 grams per kilogram of body weight per day, tailored to individual health needs and under medical supervision.

- **Individuals with Both Diabetes and Advanced Chronic Kidney Disease (CKD)**

In advanced stages of CKD, individuals should strictly control protein intake to prevent further decline in kidney function. The dietary protein intake recommended by ADA is reduced to about 0.8 grams per kilogram of body weight per day, depending on the severity of kidney disease and under healthcare professionals' guidance. For the National Kidney Foundation, the recommended daily protein intake for individuals with both diabetes and CKD stages 1-4 is 0.8 grams per kilogram of body weight. For people with diabetes and CKD stage 5 and not in dialysis RDA, the target dietary intake must be decreased to 0.6 g/kg of body weight per day.

DIABETES AND PROTEIN CHOICES

For individuals with diabetes, it is crucial to avoid ultra-processed meats and high-sodium meat products. Nutrient-dense, plant-based proteins offer fiber and antioxidants beneficial for overall health. However, exclusively plant-based diets require careful planning to avoid deficiencies in zinc, vitamin B12, calcium, and certain essential amino acids.

Nutrient Considerations in Plant-Based Diets

While plant-based diets can provide ample nutrients, it's essential to be cautious of the trend toward consuming vegan or vegetarian products designed to mimic meats and dairy. These products often fall into the category of ultra-processed foods and can contain high levels of added sugars and unhealthy additives, which do not offer the same nutritional benefits as whole, minimally processed plant foods.

UNDERSTANDING COLLAGEN: THE BODY'S BUILDING BLOCK

What is Collagen?

Collagen, constituting about 27-30% of the total protein in the human body, is a key structural component. It is essential for the integrity, elasticity, and regeneration of various tissues, including ligaments, tendons, skin, hair, nails, intervertebral discs, bones, and connective tissues. Indispensable for enhancing the durability and suppleness of our skin, collagen also facilitates smooth movement in our joints and tendons.

Main Types of Collagen:

- **Type I:** The most prevalent type, found in skin, tendons, and bones, Type I collagen is crucial for maintaining structural integrity. It helps keep these tissues firm and resilient.
- **Type II:** This type is primarily found in cartilage and bones, playing a critical role in building and supporting these connective tissues.
- **Type III:** Important for soft tissues. Type III collagen is found in muscles, blood vessels, the uterus, and intestines, providing support and elasticity.

Aging and Collagen Synthesis:

As we age, our body's ability to synthesize collagen naturally decreases. This decline begins around age 30, with an approximate reduction rate of 1% per year, and can accelerate after age 50. The reduction in collagen can lead to muscle stiffness, joint aging, wrinkles, loss of skin tone, slower wound healing, and increased fatigue.

Collagen for Diabetes:

How Much Collagen Do We Need?

The notion that collagen should make up 25-35% of our protein intake is not universally accepted. However, incorporating collagen into our diet through specific foods or supplements can offer multiple health benefits. These include enhanced skin quality, healthier joints, and increased muscle mass. Collagen supplementation might be particularly beneficial for people with diabetes as it can improve skin health, alleviate joint discomfort, stabilize blood sugar levels, and support cardiovascular health. Collagen may also benefit intestinal health, which is a concern for those with diabetes, as the condition can affect digestive processes.

Optimal Collagen Intake:

While there is no consensus on the exact percentage of daily protein intake that collagen should comprise, ensuring an adequate amount of collagen in the diet can provide significant health advantages. These benefits include improved gastrointestinal health, reduced joint pain, healthier skin, and potentially increased muscle mass. For individuals with diabetes, collagen's role in enhancing skin condition, easing joint pain, aiding blood sugar control, and supporting heart health is precious.

10

LIPIDS — ESSENTIAL MACRONUTRIENTS FOR HEALTH

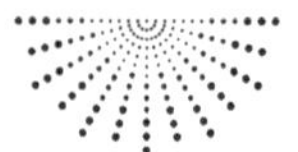

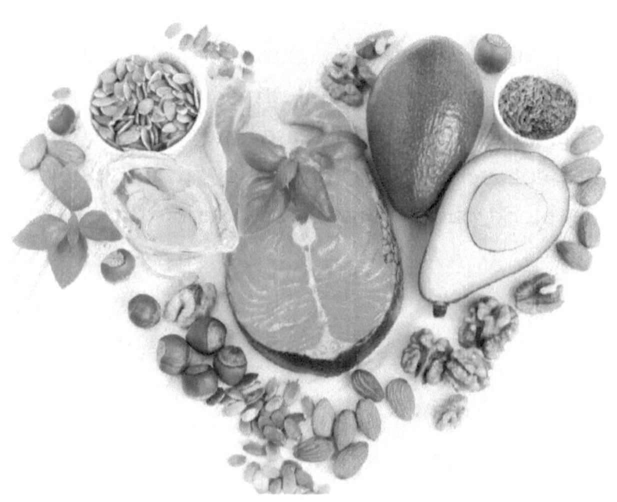

UNDERSTANDING THE ROLE OF DIETARY FATS IN HEALTH MANAGEMENT:

Dietary fats or lipids are crucial macronutrients that serve as the body's main source of stored energy and are vital for various physiological functions. They are found in foods like fats, oils, meats, dairy products, and certain plants and are primarily consumed as triglycerides. Lipids not only store energy but also contribute to cellular structure and function, regulate body temperature, and provide protection for organs. One gram of lipid provides 9 kcal of energy, which is more than double the calories provided by carbohydrates or proteins, each supplying 4 kcal per gram.

In human physiology, lipids are indispensable for maintaining cellular structure, producing sex hormones, storing energy as body fat, and regulating body temperature. They play a critical role in absorbing fat-soluble vitamins—A, D, E, and K—and enhancing foods' taste, texture, and palatability. Lipids also contribute to satiety, making them essential for a balanced diet.

Why is Fat Essential for Your Health?

Lipids are a fundamental component of a healthy diet for several reasons:

- Nutrient Absorption: Fats facilitate the absorption of fat-soluble vitamins (A, D, E, and K), vital for numerous bodily functions such as vision, bone health, antioxidant protection, and blood clotting.
- Hormone Production: Fats play a key role in synthesizing hormones that regulate various bodily processes, including growth, metabolism, and reproductive health.
- Regulation of Inflammation and Immunity: Specific fats, notably omega-3 (ω-3) fatty acids, contribute to reducing inflammation and bolstering immune function.
- Cell Health Maintenance: Fats are vital for the health of body cells. They are key components of cell membranes, impacting cell integrity and function. This includes cells in the skin and hair, contributing to their health and appearance.

CLASSIFICATION OF DIETARY FATS AND THEIR INFLUENCE ON HEALTH:

There are four primary types:

- Saturated Fat: Typically present in animal products and specific plant oils, saturated fats have a structure saturated with hydrogen atoms. Traditionally associated with heart disease and other adverse health effects, recent research indicates a more nuanced relationship with health. In diabetes and Chronic Kidney Disease (CKD), it's generally recommended to consume these fats moderately, as excessive intake can adversely affect cholesterol levels and heart health.
- Trans Fat: These are unsaturated fats that undergo chemical alteration to enhance the shelf life of food products. They are linked to adverse health outcomes, including an elevated risk of heart disease and inflammation. Trans fats are widely regarded as detrimental to health and should be minimized in the diet.
- Monounsaturated Fats (MUFAs): Present in foods such as olive oil, avocados, and select nuts, MUFAs are classified as 'healthy' fats. They promote heart health and can positively influence blood sugar control, making them especially valuable in managing diabetes.
- Polyunsaturated Fats (PUFAs): This group encompasses omega-3 and omega-6 fatty acids, which are present in fish, flaxseeds, and specific oils. Essential for numerous bodily functions, PUFAs are recognized for their anti-inflammatory properties and their support for heart and brain health. They play a crucial role in managing conditions such as diabetes and Chronic Kidney Disease.

Each type of fat plays a unique role in health, and balancing them can help manage conditions like diabetes and CKD while supporting overall well-being.

UNDERSTANDING CHOLESTEROL: ITS ROLE AND TYPES

Essential Functions of Cholesterol:

Cholesterol is a vital fat-like substance present in every body cell, essential for numerous biological functions. It forms a key component of cell membranes, enhancing their structural integrity and influencing their fluidity. Additionally, cholesterol serves as a precursor for the synthesis of several critical substances, including:

- **Vitamin D**
- **Steroid Hormones** (e.g., cortisol, aldosterone, and adrenal androgens.)
- **Sex Hormones** (e.g., testosterone, estrogens, and progesterone.)

Cholesterol also forms bile salts, crucial for digesting and absorbing fat-soluble vitamins (e.g. A, D, E, and K.)

TYPES OF CHOLESTEROL: LDL AND HDL

Cholesterol travels through the body in the form of lipoproteins, primarily as low-density lipoprotein (LDL) and high-density lipoprotein (HDL):

- **LDL Cholesterol (Low-Density Lipoprotein):** Often labeled as "bad" cholesterol, LDL carries cholesterol to cells throughout the body. High levels of LDL cholesterol are concerning because they can lead to the accumulation of plaque in arteries, heightening the risk of heart disease—risks that are elevated in individuals with diabetes and CKD.
- **HDL Cholesterol (High-Density Lipoprotein):** Known as "good" cholesterol, HDL helps transport cholesterol from the bloodstream back to the liver for excretion. Higher levels of

HDL are beneficial and linked to a diminished risk of heart disease and stroke.

CHOLESTEROL SYNTHESIS AND DIETARY IMPACT

Contrary to popular belief, the liver produces the majority of cholesterol the body needs; dietary cholesterol contributes a smaller portion to the body's total cholesterol levels. In fact, more than 85% of the cholesterol in the bloodstream is synthesized endogenously by the liver, not derived from dietary sources. Hence, dietary cholesterol typically has a minor impact on blood cholesterol levels, which is an important consideration for dietary planning, especially for individuals managing diabetes and CKD.

THE HEALTH IMPLICATIONS OF CHOLESTEROL IMBALANCE

While cholesterol is crucial for many cellular functions, an imbalance, particularly elevated LDL cholesterol levels, can be harmful. Known as hypercholesterolemia, this condition significantly increases the risk of developing premature atherosclerotic cardiovascular diseases. In the context of diabetes and CKD, it is especially critical to manage cholesterol levels as these conditions can heighten the risks associated with cholesterol imbalance.

Excess LDL cholesterol can build up on the walls of blood vessels, forming plaque and leading to health problems such as heart disease and stroke. Thus, understanding and managing cholesterol levels through lifestyle and dietary choices is essential for maintaining cardiovascular health, particularly for individuals managing chronic conditions like diabetes and CKD.

RECOMMENDED FAT TYPES FOR OPTIMAL HEALTH IN DIABETES

For individuals managing diabetes and aiming to prevent complications, focusing on consuming natural, unprocessed fat sources is crucial. Emphasizing fats high in monounsaturated and omega-3 fatty acids is particularly beneficial. These fats help manage cholesterol levels, reduce inflammation, and support cardiovascular health—key concerns for those with diabetes. In Part IV, "Dietary Guidelines and Meal Planning Principles," you'll learn how to calculate your macronutrient needs to tailor your daily intake of fats, carbohydrates, and proteins to your specific condition and lifestyle.

Healthy Fat Sources Include:

- **Avocado and Avocado Oil:** Rich in monounsaturated fats, beneficial for heart health and cholesterol management.
- **Fatty Fish (Sardines, Anchovies, Salmon):** These fish are great sources of omega-3, known for reducing inflammation and supporting heart health. They may also positively influence blood glucose levels.
- **Olives and Olive Oil:** Packed with MUFAs and antioxidants, olive oil is an effective heart-healthy choice that helps stabilize blood sugar levels.
- **• Nuts and Nut Oils (Macadamias, Almonds, Brazil Nuts, Hazelnuts, Pecans):** These nuts provide a balanced blend of monounsaturated and polyunsaturated fats, which are advantageous for both heart health and overall nutritional well-being.
- **Flaxseeds and Flaxseed Oil:** These are good sources of alpha-linolenic acid (ALA), a type of omega-3 renowned for its anti-inflammatory properties and blood sugar control benefits.
- **Walnuts and Walnut Oil:** These are good sources of omega-3 fatty acids, which improve endothelial function and are crucial for cardiovascular health.

- **Chia Seeds:** These kind of seeds are packed with omega-3, fiber, and antioxidants, supporting heart health and blood glucose management.
- **Sunflower Seeds and Sunflower Oil:** They Provide vitamin E and healthy fats, though they should be consumed in moderation due to their higher omega-6 content.
- **Extra Virgin Olive Oil:** Abundant in antioxidants and monounsaturated fats, it proves advantageous in managing heart health and conditions such as diabetes and chronic kidney disease.

11
ESSENTIAL MICRONUTRIENTS IN DIABETES DIET

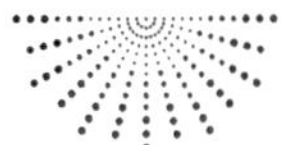

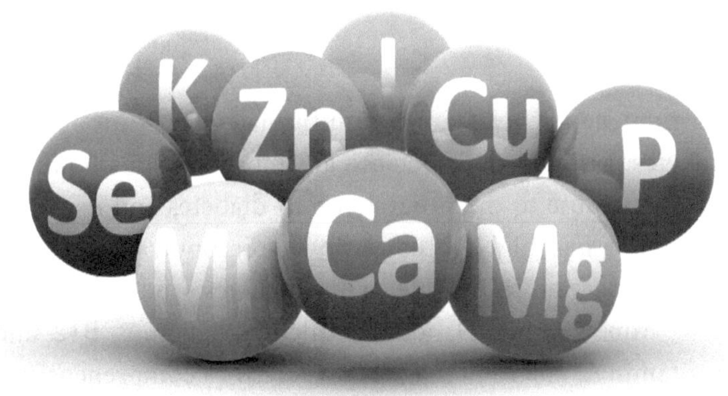

UNDERSTANDING MICRONUTRIENTS IN HEALTH MAINTENANCE

Micronutrients, including essential minerals and vitamins, are crucial for human health, regulating vital physiological functions throughout life. Despite being needed in tiny amounts, they play a significant role in maintaining overall well-being. A deficiency in minerals or vitamins can lead to serious health issues, especially for individuals managing chronic conditions such as diabetes, hypertension, and early-stage Chronic Kidney Disease (CKD).

Significance of Micronutrients in Metabolic Functions:

Micronutrients are vital for numerous metabolic reactions, supporting metabolism and tissue function. Deficiencies in micronutrients can lead to various symptoms, including:

- Fatigue and sleep disturbances
- Mood changes and irritability
- Cognitive impairments
- Increased stress levels
- Paleness
- Digestive issues
- Chronic headaches
- Muscle tension
- Heart palpitations

Micronutrient deficiencies are a significant concern for individuals with diabetes, as these deficiencies can impact various bodily functions and contribute to the progression of diabetes and its complications. Research has highlighted various micronutrient deficiencies commonly observed in people with diabetes, including but not limited to iron, vitamin D, iodine, calcium, vitamins B12 and B9 (folate), vitamin A, zinc, and magnesium. Here's a comprehensive list:

- **Iron:** Indispensable for oxygen transport in the blood and for preventing anemia.
- **Vitamin D:** Crucial for bone health, immune function, and regulating calcium absorption.
- **Iodine:** Indispensable for the production of thyroid hormones, which regulate metabolism.
- **Calcium:** Key for maintaining bone structure and function as well as muscle and nerve function.

- **Vitamins B12 and B9 (Folate):** Important for neurological function, DNA synthesis, red blood cell formation, etc.
- **Vitamin A:** Vital for vision, immune health, and skin integrity.
- **Zinc:** Important in immune function, wound healing, and DNA synthesis.
- **Magnesium:** Essential mineral involved in over 350 biochemical reactions in the body (e.g., energy production, nerve function, and muscle relaxation.)
- **Vitamin C:** Important for immune function, skin health, and antioxidant protection.
- **Vitamin E:** This fat-soluble vitamin is a potent antioxidant. It has numerous essential roles (cell protection from damage, immune function support, etc.)
- **Selenium:** This essential trace element is critical in human health (e.g., metabolism, thyroid function, antioxidant properties.)

MICRONUTRIENTS IN DIABETES MANAGEMENT:

Managing diabetes can benefit from careful attention to micronutrient levels. Emerging research suggests that certain micronutrients may have therapeutic benefits in managing Type 2 Diabetes Mellitus (T2DM):

- **Vitamin D:** Studies indicate that vitamin D might improve glycemic control and potentially reduce the risk of diabetes-related complications. It may enhance insulin sensitivity and reduce inflammation.
- **Vitamin K:** There is increasing interest in vitamin K's role in vascular health, which may impact diabetes-related complications. It's hypothesized that vitamin K could aid in improving insulin sensitivity and reduce inflammation.
- **Magnesium:** Magnesium is known to play a role in glucose

metabolism. Adequate magnesium levels are associated with enhanced blood sugar control and a lower risk of T2DM.

- **Chromium:** Chromium is believed to enhance insulin sensitivity. It's crucial to be cautious when taking chromium supplements alongside diabetes medications, as it can lower blood sugar levels. This increases the risk of hypoglycemia, particularly when used with insulin, metformin, or other oral medications that improve insulin sensitivity or increase beta-cell insulin release.

PART III
THE LOW GL DIABETES DIET: A SUSTAINABLE STRATEGY FOR ENHANCED BLOOD SUGAR MANAGEMENT

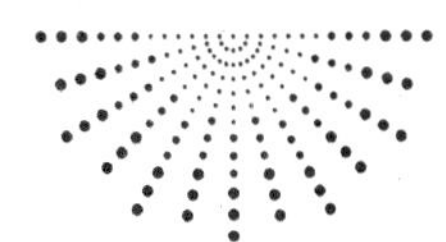

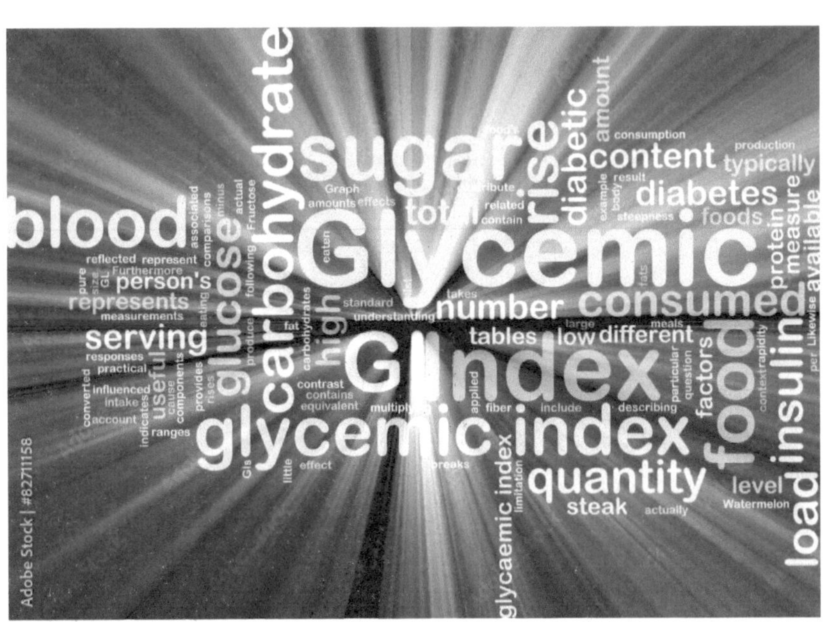

12

THE LOW-GL DIET: UNDERSTANDING THE CONCEPT AND REAPING THE BENEFITS

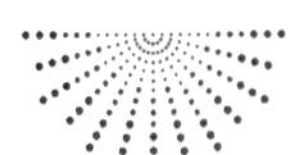

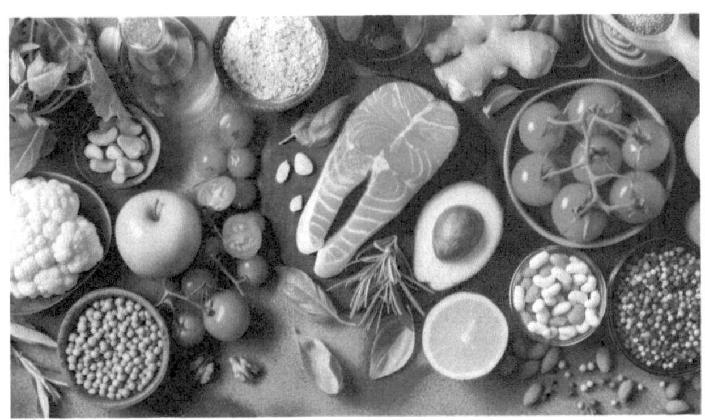

The GL Diabetes Diet: A Comprehensive Approach to Diabetes Management

Diabetes management strategies have traditionally centered on optimizing key markers like glycated hemoglobin (HbA1c), fasting plasma glucose (FPG), and postprandial glucose (PPG), as recommended by the American Diabetes Association. The low glycemic index & load diet, a scientifically backed eating plan, has evolved significantly from its initial focus on assessing and ranking foods based on their glycemic impact. It has transformed into a comprehensive dietary approach, integrating not just the glycemic effect of foods but also considering the quality and quantity of carbohydrates they contain, promoting balanced and healthy eating habits.

This dietary approach, as promoted in this book, goes beyond just assessing the glycemic impact. It includes practical elements tailored explicitly for diabetes management, such as portion control with a standard serving size of 15 grams of carbohydrates, as per the CDC guidelines. It aligns with the 2020-2025 Dietary Guidelines for Americans, covering aspects that indirectly affect blood sugar levels.

Type 2 diabetes is marked by persistent hyperglycemia and insulin resistance, which are pivotal in the onset of diabetic complications. Effective management of T2D, therefore, must target two primary goals: reducing hyperglycemia and reversing insulin resistance. The Low GL Diabetes Diet helps achieve the former by minimizing sharp blood glucose spikes. The latter goal can be addressed by enhancing diet quality, promoting weight loss, practicing intermittent fasting, and incorporating dietary elements like Extra Virgin Olive Oil (EVOO). This diet, which is the focus of this book, emerges from this dual consideration. As you will learn, it is straightforward and evidence-based, equipping you with essential knowledge for effective carbohydrate management and improved blood glucose control.

The disparity in health outcomes between individuals who adhere to the Low GL Diabetes Diet principles, even at a basic level, versus those solely focused on carbohydrate counting, is significant. Those who follow the GL principles generally achieve better overall diabetes control. They select foods that release sugar into the bloodstream slowly, leading to more stable blood sugar levels, lower A1C levels, and more favorable lipid profiles. Conversely, those who equate all carbohydrates and rely only on carbohydrate counting often experience poorer diabetes control, higher A1C levels, and less favorable lipid profiles.

Since the 2000s, I have consistently encouraged patients to consider both the glycemic index and carbohydrate content of foods. This recommendation is aligned with the guidance provided by many endocrinologists. To facilitate this, I compiled a comprehensive list of common foods, detailing their glycemic index, portion size, carbohydrate content, and glycemic load. This resource has proven invaluable for thousands of patients, helping them stabilize their blood sugar levels and improve their A1C by opting for lower GI foods over higher GI options.

Understanding the Consequences of Elevated Blood Sugar Levels on the Body

I have intentionally chosen to delve into the effects of high blood sugar on the body in this chapter to underscore the direct connection between diet and health outcomes. The foods you consume significantly influence your blood sugar, which in turn affects your body, blood vessels, and organs. This direct link from diet to blood sugar and subsequently to the health of your body systems is critical to better understanding and grasping these risks. Let's explore the mechanisms at play:

- **Vascular Damage and Glycation of Proteins:** High blood sugar can damage the walls of small blood vessels, leading to complications. This damage is partly due to glycation, where glucose binds to proteins, forming Advanced Glycation Endproducts (AGEs). AGEs damage the structure and function of proteins, reducing elasticity and impairing vascular function.
- **Nerve Damage and Endothelial Dysfunction:** Elevated glucose levels can interfere with nerve signals and the health of blood vessels, leading to neuropathy. In the blood vessels, high glucose damages endothelial cells, impairing their ability to produce nitric oxide, which is crucial for vessel dilation. This can increase the risk of hypertension and atherosclerosis.
- **Organ Complications and Inflammatory**

Response: Chronic high blood sugar contributes to severe conditions affecting the heart, kidneys, eyes, and brain. It also activates inflammatory pathways, such as NF-κB, producing inflammatory cytokines and attracting immune cells. This exacerbates vascular damage and the development of atherosclerotic plaque.

- **Oxidative Stress:** Hyperglycemia augments the production of Reactive Oxygen Species (ROS) in blood vessels, damaging the endothelium. High blood sugar also impairs antioxidant defenses, increasing oxidative stress.
- **Hyperglycemia-Induced Hypercoagulability:** Elevated blood sugar alters the properties of blood, increasing the clotting tendency due to changes in platelet function, clotting factors, and blood flow dynamics.
- **Vascular Smooth Muscle Cell Dysfunction:** Elevated glucose levels promote unusual growth and movement of vascular smooth muscle cells, causing the walls of vessels to thicken and the openings to narrow, thus obstructing blood flow.
- **Lipid Abnormalities:** Diabetes often involves changes in lipid metabolism, leading to higher levels of LDL and triglycerides, contributing to vascular damage.

Recognizing these mechanisms underscores the critical need for controlled blood sugar levels. The low GL diabetes diet offers a practical and adaptable approach to achieving this, providing a wide range of food choices with fewer restrictions than more stringent or extreme diets, such as high-fat, low-carb regimens, or the more permissive yet limited approach of carb counting.

Introducing the Glycemic Index Concept: Postprandial (After-Meal) Responses

The Glycemic Index (GI) concept is intimately linked with the body's postprandial responses—the physiological changes that occur after eating. This section explores these responses, setting the stage for understanding the concepts of GI and Glycemic Load (GL).

Postprandial Blood Glucose Responses: The Foundation of the GI Concept

Postprandial responses, which have been studied extensively in the fields of physiology, endocrinology, and biochemistry, are vital for understanding how our body reacts to different foods. Significant milestones such as the discovery of secretin by William M. Bayliss and Ernest H. Starling in 1902, and insulin by Frederick Banting and Charles Best in 1921, have been pivotal in advancing our knowledge about how blood sugar is regulated after meals, especially in the context of diabetes management.

Immediate Response to Food Intake:

- **Carbohydrate Absorption:** When we consume food, the carbohydrates present are metabolized into glucose and absorbed into the bloodstream. This process leads to an increase in blood glucose levels, the extent of which is influenced by the type of carbohydrates consumed, as well as the meal's fiber, fat, and protein content.

The Body's Insulin Response:

- **Insulin Release and Function:** The pancreas secretes insulin in response to increased glucose levels. This hormone plays a crucial role in permitting glucose uptake by cells for energy use or storage, thereby helping to decrease blood glucose levels.

THE GLYCEMIC INDEX: A CRUCIAL TOOL IN DIABETES MANAGEMENT

Introduced in 1981 by Dr. David Jenkins and his research team at the University of Toronto, the Glycemic Index (GI) marked a pivotal moment in our comprehension of how carbohydrate-rich foods influence blood glucose levels. This innovative concept transformed our dietary understanding, providing a refined insight into the metabolic response to different foods. By assessing the rate at which foods elevate blood sugar levels relative to pure glucose, the GI offers a valuable tool for individuals seeking to manage their blood sugar and optimize their dietary choices. Dr. Jenkins' groundbreaking work laid the foundation for further research into the complex interplay between diet, metabolism, and health outcomes.

FACTORS INFLUENCING GLYCEMIC RESPONSES

- **Starch Composition and Properties:** Including digestibility, amylose/amylopectin ratio, and changes due to cooking (gelatinization) and cooling (retrogradation).
- **Dietary Fiber Content:** Food type and amount of fiber can significantly affect the glycemic response.
- **Types of Sugar:** Different sugars in foods can impact blood glucose levels differently.
- **Other Influential Factors:** Insulin response, protein content, food processing techniques, particle size, fat content, acidity, storage conditions, and harvest time.

GLYCEMIC INDEX CATEGORIZATION

The Glycemic Index (GI) categorizes Carbohydrates and the foods containing them based on their post-meal effects on blood glucose levels. This classification system divides foods into three main categories: **high-GI (GI ≥ 70)**, **medium-GI (GI between 56 and 69)**, and

low-GI (GI ≤ 55). These categories reflect the varying rates at which carbohydrates are digested and absorbed by the body after consumption. Foods with a high GI value undergo rapid digestion and absorption, causing a quick surge in blood glucose and insulin levels. On the contrary, low-GI foods undergo digestion and absorption at a slower pace, leading to a gradual and steady augmentation in blood glucose levels, as illustrated in the following figure:

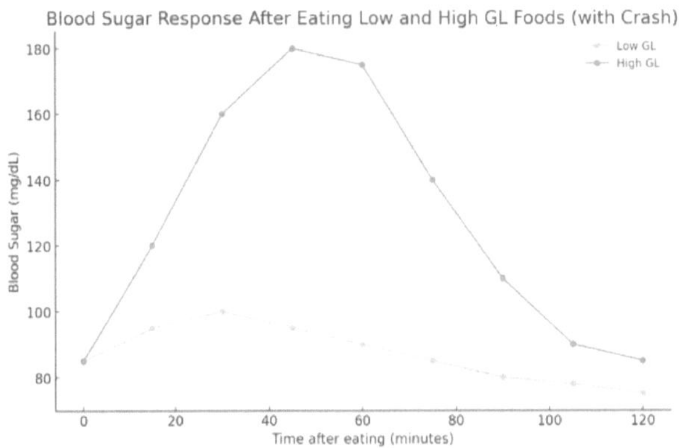

To clarify this concept, let's examine the examples of an apple and a ripe banana calibrated to have the same net carbohydrate content. By comparing these two fruits, which have different glycemic index values despite similar carbohydrate content, we can illustrate how the GI concept elucidates the physiological impacts of various foods on blood sugar levels.

Example 1: Apple

- **Food:** Apple (1 medium, approximately 182g)
- **Net Carbohydrates:** 21 grams
- **Glycemic Index (GI):** 36

This example illustrates that a medium-sized apple, which weighs around 182 grams and contains 21 grams of net carbohydrates, has a

GI of 36. This low GI value indicates that the apple will have a low impact on blood sugar levels compared to pure glucose. To determine how many grams of pure glucose would have a similar effect on blood sugar as this apple, we use the following formula:

$$\text{Equivalent glucose amount} = \left(\frac{\text{Net carbohydrates}}{100}\right) \times \text{GI}$$

Substituting in the values:

$$\text{Equivalent glucose amount} = \left(\frac{21\ \text{grams}}{100}\right) \times 36$$

$$\text{Equivalent glucose amount} \approx 7.56\ \text{grams}$$

Equivalent glucose amount≈7.56 grams

- Thus, **consuming a medium-sized apple similarly affects blood sugar as consuming approximately 7.56 grams of pure glucose.**

Example 2: Ripe Banana

- Food: Banana (1 small, approximately 85g)
- Net Carbohydrates: 21 grams
- Glycemic Index: 75

In this example, a small ripe banana with the same net carbohydrate content as the apple (21 grams) has a GI of 75, which is significantly higher. This suggests a greater impact on blood sugar levels. Calculating the equivalent glucose effect:

$$\text{Equivalent glucose amount} = \left(\frac{21 \text{ grams}}{100}\right) \times 75$$

$$\text{Equivalent glucose amount} \approx 15.75 \text{ grams}$$

- Thus, **consuming a small banana similarly affects blood sugar as consuming approximately 15.75 grams of pure glucose.**

These two examples demonstrate how the GI can be used to categorize foods as having low, medium, or high impacts on blood sugar and make more precise comparisons within the same category. For instance, even though both the apple and banana might fall into the same broad category based on their net carbohydrate content, the apple's lower GI value means it has a lesser impact on blood sugar levels.

LIMITATIONS OF THE GLYCEMIC INDEX CONCEPT

The glycemic index provides insight into how foods can impact blood sugar, yet it is not without its drawbacks:

- **Portion Sizes Not Accounted For**: GI measures the impact of a standard amount of carbohydrate on the blood sugar in foods, not considering the quantity consumed. Glycemic load (GL) complements GI by factoring in serving size to reflect a food's effect on blood sugar accurately.
- **Food Preparation and Combination Effects**: The GI of a food can fluctuate based on its preparation method. For example, pasta cooked to the al dente stage typically exhibits a lower GI compared to when it is cooked to the point of being overdone. Additionally, the combination of foods—such as incorporating fats or proteins—can modify the glycemic response to a carbohydrate-rich meal.
- **Neglect of Nutrient Content**: GI does not reflect the

nutritional richness of foods; some high GI foods are nutrient-dense, while some low GI foods offer little nutritional value. Relying solely on GI could mislead people about the healthiness of their food choices.

- **Limited Scope for Non-Carbohydrate Foods**: Foods without carbohydrates, like pure meats and oils, lack a GI value, which can lead to confusion when planning a balanced diet.
- **Inconsistencies in Food GI Values**: Variations in GI can occur even within the same type of food due to differences in ripeness, processing, and brand, leading to inconsistencies and potential confusion for those trying to adhere to GI guidelines.

These limitations emphasize the necessity for a balanced approach. While GI may benefit diet management, relying solely on it can lead to overconsumption of low-GI foods, resulting in overeating, potential nutritional imbalances, and inconsistent blood sugar control.

THE LOW-GL DIABETES DIET APPROACH

The Low-GL Diabetes Diet addresses the Glycemic Index limitations by utilizing the Glycemic Load concept, **which considers both the quality and quantity of ingested foods**. This approach aligns with authoritative dietary guidelines, such as those from the 2020-2025 Dietary Guidelines for Americans, and incorporates principles of the Mediterranean diet and a balanced diet. It aims to correct the inconsistencies inherent in the GI system.

For example, mango, with a low GI of 54, is considered acceptable for unrestricted consumption under the GI framework. At the same time, watermelon, with a higher GI of 72, is typically recommended to be avoided. **According to GI guidelines, one could consume three cups of mango, introducing 84 grams of carbohydrates** into their diet. However, they **should avoid even ½ cup of watermelon, which contains only 5.8 grams of carbohydrates.**

This guideline presents a significant issue for individuals with diabetes and even for those without the condition; such eating patterns could potentially be harmful. Furthermore, the **GI-focused eating pattern may exclude nutrient-rich foods like watermelon based on their GI while encouraging the consumption of lower-quality foods if they have a low GI**. The striking example of margarine made with artificial trans fats, which may have a low GI, illustrates this flaw.

By basing the diet on the GL framework and integrating the 2020-2025 Recommended Dietary Allowances (RDAs) and Mediterranean diet principles, ***the Low-GL Diabetes Diet rectifies these inconsistencies and offers a powerful dietary approach for diabetes management.***

THE GLYCEMIC LOAD FOR ENHANCED BLOOD SUGAR MANAGEMENT

Harvard University researchers developed the Glycemic Load (GL) as a more precise metric for managing blood sugar. GL addresses the limitations of the Glycemic Index (GI), which does not consider portion size. It combines the GI value with the actual carbohydrate content of a standard serving, offering a more accurate depiction of how foods affect blood sugar levels. This is particularly crucial for managing diabetes and preventing blood sugar spikes.

Unlike GI, which lacks direct physiological relevance, GL values represent the blood sugar response to consuming one gram of glucose —equating 1 GL to 1 gram of pure glucose. This concrete measure accounts for both the quality and quantity of carbohydrates, making GL a superior tool for diabetes management compared to GI.

GL allows individuals to better manage portion sizes, helping to avoid overconsumption of carbohydrates and the resultant blood sugar spikes and crashes. The low-GL diabetes diet, based on this concept, supports a varied and nutritious diet by promoting balanced portion sizes and minimizing the risks associated with excessive carbohydrate intake.

The Glycemic Load system provides a robust way for people to classify foods according to their impact on blood sugar levels. Here's a detailed outline of the Glycemic Load rankings:

- **Low GL:** Foods that score 10 or less on the GL scale are considered to have a minimal impact on blood sugar. These are ideal choices for maintaining stable glucose levels throughout the day.
- **Medium GL:** A GL score between 11 and 19 indicates a moderate effect on blood sugar. Such foods can be included occasionally in the diet with consideration of overall carbohydrate intake and timing relative to activity levels.
- **High GL:** Foods with a GL score of 20 or more significantly impact blood sugar. They must be avoided or consumed less frequently in very smaller portions, especially for individuals focused on strict blood sugar control.

ADDITIONAL CONSIDERATIONS:

Glycemic Load (GL) of Combined Meals: The GL of a combined meal is the sum of the GLs of each component. Even if individual foods have low GL values, combining them can result in a higher overall GL, which may affect blood sugar levels differently.

Recommendations on Added Sugars Intake: The CDC, American Diabetes Association (ADA), and other authoritative organizations suggest that individuals with diabetes limit added sugar / free sugar intake to no more than 10% of total daily calories, corresponding to 50 grams of added sugars per day, which translates into a maximum of 50 GL per day.

Impact of Food Processing: The processing and cooking methods applied to foods can affect their glycemic load. Highly processed foods tend to have higher GL values than whole, minimally processed foods.

Balancing Carbohydrates with Proteins and Fats: Combining carbohydrates with proteins and healthy fats can mitigate the glycemic impact of meals.

Timing of Meals and Snacks: Spacing meals and snacks evenly throughout the day aids maintain stable blood sugar levels and prevents significant fluctuations. Each meal should incorporate a balanced combination of carbohydrates, proteins, and fats to promote sustained energy and feelings of fullness while managing glycemic load.

Physical Activity: Regular physical activity enhances insulin sensitivity and blood sugar control, mitigating the effects of high-glycemic foods. Integrating exercise into your routine is crucial for managing glycemic load and promoting better metabolic health.

WATERMELON: A PRACTICAL ILLUSTRATION OF THE GLYCEMIC INDEX AND LOAD

Watermelon is an excellent example of the practical application of the Glycemic Index (GI) and Glycemic Load (GL) concepts. Despite its high GI of 72, watermelon has a low glycemic load of approximately 6, mainly due to its modest carbohydrate content.

A typical serving size of 120 grams (equivalent to about two thin slices, or ¼ of a circle edge each), or one cup (150 grams) of diced watermelon, comprises about 9 grams of natural sugar and 11.5 grams of carbohydrates. This is less than the standard recommended carbohydrate serving of 15 grams.

Therefore, the glycemic load of a single serving of watermelon is approximately 6, categorizing it as low. This implies that watermelon can be a more favorable option for blood sugar management than its GI value alone might indicate.

Understanding the Postprandial Impact of Watermelon

When you consume a 150-gram serving of diced watermelon, your body quickly absorbs the 9 grams of natural sugars and 11.5 grams of carbohydrates. The high GI of watermelon indicates that these carbohydrates will be rapidly released into the bloodstream, aligning with the fruit's nutritional profile. This is because watermelon has a low fiber content of only 0.6 grams per 150-gram serving and is primarily composed of simple sugars (sucrose, fructose, and glucose), along with minimal protein (0.9 g) and virtually no fat.

As you eat watermelon, the sugars break down, starting in your mouth and then continuing into your digestive tract, where they are absorbed into your bloodstream as glucose. This process elevates your blood sugar level, prompting your pancreas to release insulin. However, due to the low glycemic load of watermelon, the magnitude of this blood sugar rise is small (9 grams of net carb).

In contrast, consuming high-GI and high-GL foods would result in a more significant blood sugar spike.

Therefore, relying on the GL of foods like watermelon helps make informed dietary choices. This knowledge allows for including various fruits and foods in the diet while maintaining good glycemic control.

BUCKWHEAT SPAGHETTI: A PRACTICAL ILLUSTRATION OF THE IMPACT OF COOKING TIME

Initial Glycemic Index (GI) and Glycemic Load (GL) of Buckwheat Spaghetti:

Buckwheat spaghetti, when cooked to yield a portion of 70 grams (approximately ½ cup cooked), has a Glycemic Index (GI) of roughly

45 and a Glycemic Load (GL) of 9.5. These values categorize the spaghetti as having both a low GI and a low GL, which is favorable for blood sugar management, as foods with a GL of 10 or less are categorized low.

Effect of Cooking Duration on GL:

The cooking duration influences the Glycemic Index of buckwheat spaghetti. Cooking the spaghetti al dente, which means it's still firm to the bite, tends to keep the GI relatively stable, close to its original value (GI of 45). This stability is due to the less broken-down state of carbohydrates, which slows digestion. However, cooking the spaghetti for a shorter duration, such as 5 minutes, may slightly increase the GI, but not significantly (GI of 54). In contrast, cooking the spaghetti for an extended period, such as 12 minutes or more, can considerably increase the GI. This increase might push the GI value above 55, transitioning it from a low to a medium GI because longer cooking times break down the carbohydrates more thoroughly, making them easier to digest and absorb, thereby raising the GI.

Changes in GL with Cooking Time:

The cooking duration may also affect the Glycemic Load (GL) along with the GI. Since GL is a measure that considers both the carbohydrate content and the GI, any increase in the GI mechanically elevates the GL. It is common for the GL to shift from low to medium if the GI increases significantly due to prolonged cooking times for pasta and rice.

Salmon, Herring, and Tuna: Understanding the Impact of Cooking Preparation

Salmon, herring, and tuna are excellent choices for a diabetic diet due to their high omega-3 content, which can reduce inflammation in blood cells and help improve cholesterol levels. While fish and seafood are generally beneficial due to their lean protein, omega-3 fatty acids, and minimal carbohydrate content, it's essential to recognize that cooking methods can significantly influence their Glycemic Index (GI) and Glycemic Load (GL).

Unsuitable Cooking Methods in the Context of the Low GL Diabetes Diet:

• **Battered and Fried Fish:** Fish, naturally low in unhealthy fats and free of carbohydrates, becomes less beneficial when breaded and fried. The batter, usually a mixture of water, flour, and seasonings, can add significant carbohydrates and increase the GI. Battering can contribute up to 20% of the final product, altering its nutritional profile.

• **Breaded and Fried Fish:** Similar to battered fish, breaded and fried fish, though naturally low in fats and carbs, becomes less healthy when prepared this way. The breading, typically made from refined grains, adds extra carbohydrates. Furthermore, the frying process increases the calorie content and may contribute to insulin resistance and the formation of Advanced Glycation End-products.

• **Breaded and Fried Seafood:** Breaded and fried seafood items, like shrimp or calamari, follow the same pattern. Due to the breading and frying process, they are high in unhealthy fats, calories, and refined grains. This preparation method can lead to blood sugar spikes and worsen inflammation.

It is essential to note that the raw GI of fish and seafood is virtually zero. However, preparation methods like frying can substantially alter their nutritional value, leading to increased caloric intake and potential negative impacts on blood sugar management and inflammation. Therefore, for individuals following the GL Diabetes Diet, particularly those managing diabetes, selecting the proper preparation methods for fish and seafood is key to maintaining their health benefits.

Bananas, Apples, Pears: Understanding the Impact of Ripeness on the Glycemic Index and Load

Bananas, apples, and pears provide excellent examples to illustrate how ripeness influences the Glycemic Index (GI) and Glycemic Load (GL) of fruits—considerations crucial for diabetes management. These fruits, rich in nutrients such as vitamins, minerals, and fiber, offer health benefits. However, their generally higher carbohydrate content than vegetables requires careful management, especially for those with diabetes. This is where understanding the GL becomes particularly important.

Comparing Fruit Servings and Ripeness in GI and GL Analysis

A standard 15-gram carbohydrate serving of fruit—like a medium apple, small banana, or small pear—may seem equivalent at first glance. However, ripeness significantly alters their GI and GL values. For instance, while unripe bananas have a low GI of around 51, partially ripe ones have a moderate GI of 62, and fully ripe bananas can have a high GI, reaching up to 75. Similar changes in GI occur in other fruits as they ripen.

The Role of Ripeness in GI and GL Variation:

Mature Green (Unripe) Stage: Here, fruits contain more starch and less simple sugar. The higher starch content produces a firmer texture and less sweetness, often accompanied by a more acidic or bitter taste.

Partial Ripe Stage: As fruits ripen, enzymes break down complex carbohydrates like starch into simpler sugars such as sucrose, glucose, and fructose. This enzymatic activity increases the fruit's sweetness and makes its texture softer and juicier.

Fully Ripe Stage: In this final stage, the starch-to-sugar conversion is nearly complete, with high levels of simple sugars contributing to the fruit's maximum sweetness and soft texture. The flavor and aroma are also fully developed at this stage.

This transformation, resulting from sugar accumulation from the plant and the conversion of stored carbohydrates, is key to the fruit's flavor development, texture, and nutritional value.

The GI Rise With Ripening:

Unripe bananas have a low GI (around 51), which increases to a moderate level (62) in partially ripe bananas, and reaches a high GI (up to 75) when fully ripe.

Other fruits exhibit similar trends, though the extent varies. For example, apples typically maintain a low GI even when fully ripe, increasing only from 36 to 51 in overripe stages.

Fruits on the higher end of the low-GI scale may shift into the medium-GI category as they ripen, impacting their suitability within a GL-focused diet.

Understanding how ripeness affects the GI and GL of fruits like bananas, apples, and pears allows for including a variety of fruits in the diet while maintaining optimal glycemic control.

13
THE 15 CORE PRINCIPLES

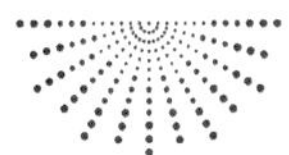

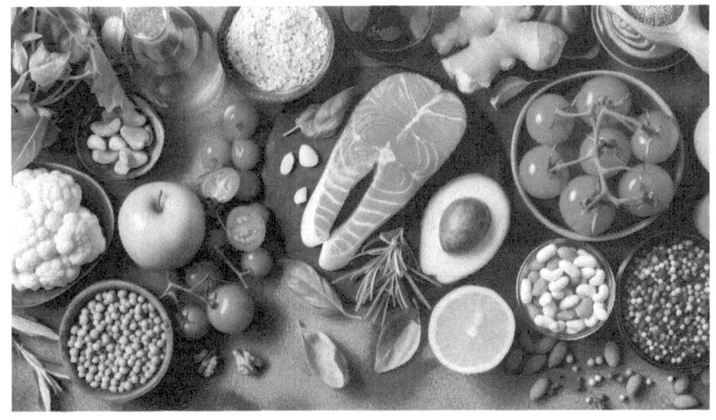

THE LOW GL DIABETES DIET: A PRACTICAL APPROACH TO MANAGING DIABETES

The Low GL Diabetes Diet is based on 15 fundamental principles designed to simplify adherence to healthy eating habits. These principles specifically address the challenges faced by individuals managing diabetes. They also cover key dietary concerns, including the risks associated with processed foods, the impact of high glycemic index foods on health and weight, and the consequences of consuming excess sugar and sodium.

These principles, developed to be practical and comprehensive, are crafted to enhance both diabetes care and general well-being. They are formatted to be user-friendly and easily adaptable, suitable for use as flashcards, reminder cards, or quick reference notes. This approach stems from my experiences with patients whose journeys with diabetes have underscored the need for actionable, straightforward guidance.

These 15 core principles are not merely theoretical; they are actionable steps born from extensive knowledge and experience. They promote a proactive, action-driven approach to diabetes management. As you progress through each chapter, you will find the Low GL Diabetes Diet increasingly familiar and easy to integrate into your daily routine.

Designed to save time and effort in diet planning, these principles facilitate effective meal planning across the five food groups and culminate in a comprehensive resource found in the final volume—the GI, GL, and net Carb counter for over 2,000 commonly consumed foods. This exhaustive, easy-to-follow approach has proven effective in managing diabetes, helping you confidently navigate your dietary needs.

PRINCIPLE 1: EAT LOW-GLYCEMIC LOAD FOODS

The Low Glycemic Load Diabetes Diet centers on low-GL foods, essential for aiding weight loss, enhancing blood sugar management, and improving overall health. This diet prioritizes whole and minimally processed foods, aligning with the latest dietary guidelines to ensure a well-rounded diet. Detailed guidelines about nutritional recommendations, macronutrient distribution, and meal planning principles are provided in Part IV, "Dietary Guidelines and Meal Planning Principles."

Principle 2: Increase Olive Oil Consumption

Extra-virgin olive oil (EVOO) is a beneficial addition to the Low GL Diabetes Diet, thanks to its content of monounsaturated fatty acids. These healthy fats help improve cholesterol levels, reduce inflammation, and decrease heart disease risk. EVOO is a main component of the Mediterranean diet, known for its positive effects on diabetes management.

Research strongly supports the inclusion of extra-virgin olive oil in the diet to help lower blood sugar levels, bad LDL cholesterol, and triglycerides. Not only does EVOO aid in weight loss, but it also plays a role in preventing and managing diabetes. The anti-diabetic properties of EVOO are enhanced with higher daily consumption, with studies suggesting a minimum of four tablespoons per day to achieve its antioxidant and anti-diabetic effects.

When integrated into the Low GL Diabetes Diet, EVOO can contribute to weight loss and better blood sugar control. Studies indicate that diets high in monounsaturated fats like EVOO can lead to more significant weight loss and improved insulin sensitivity than diets high in carbohydrates.

In the upcoming chapter titled "Macronutrient Distribution for Your Diabetes Diet," you'll discover the importance of balancing your daily intake of carbohydrates, fats, and proteins. You'll learn that carbohydrates should make up 45-50% of your daily caloric intake, leaving 50-55% divided between fats and proteins. Specifically, fats should constitute 25-30% of your total calorie consumption, emphasizing monounsaturated and polyunsaturated fatty acids. EVOO should comprise a significant portion of this fat intake, leveraging its monounsaturated fats to the fullest extent for your health.

PRINCIPLE 3: LIMIT ADDED SUGAR INTAKE

In the low GL Diabetes Diet, a pivotal focus is placed on minimizing the intake of added sugars. These sugars often masquerade under various aliases like corn syrup, fructose, and glucose, stealthily infiltrating our daily diet. The pervasiveness of these hidden sugars, particularly in processed foods and sweetened beverages, poses a significant challenge for individuals managing diabetes, as they can dramatically impact blood sugar levels.

Fructose, commonly incorporated into foods such as high fructose corn syrup (HFCS), stands out for its potential to exacerbate diabetes-related metabolic issues. Developed from corn starch, HFCS is found in a wide range of food products, often chosen for its ability to enhance taste and consistency. It typically comprises 42% to 55% fructose and has become a staple ingredient in the food industry. However, the body's response to fructose, especially when produced internally due to diabetes or high-sugar diets, can lead to various health concerns.

The high Glycemic Index (GI) of common added sugars like sucrose and HFCS is a major area of concern in the Low GL Diabetes Diet. These sugars rapidly enter the bloodstream, causing swift and significant spikes in blood glucose levels. Regular consumption of these high-GI sugars can lead to increased blood sugar levels and heighten the risk of insulin resistance, thus impeding effective diabetes management.

The fructose metabolism, primarily occurring in the liver, can induce several metabolic complications. It can increase triglyceride production, elevating the risk of heart disease and contributing to insulin resistance. Excessive fructose intake is also linked to the onset of non-alcoholic fatty liver disease (NAFLD). Additionally, fructose's lack of impact on regulating hunger hormones like insulin and leptin can increase calorie intake and weight gain, further complicating diabetes management.

PRINCIPLE 4: REDUCE SODIUM INTAKE

In the context of the GL Diabetes Diet, managing sodium intake is more than just a dietary guideline; it's a critical component in comprehensive diabetes management. This approach is not only about controlling diabetes effectively but also about addressing the heightened risk of severe health complications that arise from the combination of diabetes and hypertension. The primary aim of an effective diabetes diet is to prevent or halt the progression of diabetes-related severe complications, such as chronic kidney disease (CKD), cardiovascular disease, nerve damage, and eye damage.

Given the fact that Individuals with diabetes have a twofold increased likelihood of developing high blood pressure as those without, managing hypertension is a strategic move to minimize the compounded damage to blood vessels and organs caused by both high blood sugar and high blood pressure.

Looking at the average American diet, we find a worrying trend: it typically contains over 3,400 milligrams (mg) of sodium daily, significantly surpassing the recommended limit. The Dietary Guidelines for Americans suggest limiting sodium intake to less than 2,300 mg per day, a benchmark that is crucial in the GL Diabetes Diet as well. This threshold is not arbitrary; it's grounded in the need to address the widespread prevalence of hypertension—a condition that was a primary or contributing cause of approximately 691,095 deaths in the U.S. in 2021 alone. To visualize this sodium limit, consider one level teaspoon of table salt containing about 2,300 mg.

For individuals with both diabetes and hypertension, the stakes are even higher. They face a 40% increased risk of heart attack and stroke compared to those with diabetes alone. This statistic underscores the importance of sodium restriction as a critical strategy in the Low GL Diabetes Diet.

Moreover, for individuals with diabetes who also have chronic kidney disease (CKD), particularly in stages 3-5, sodium restriction becomes even more stringent. This is due to the kidneys' decreased ability to effectively filter and balance sodium and other electrolytes.

PRINCIPLE 5: INCORPORATE POLYPHENOL-RICH FOODS

Adding polyphenol-rich foods to your diet is wise for anyone following the Low GL Diabetes Diet. Polyphenols, powerful antioxidants in many plants, are known for boosting health in several ways. They can reduce inflammation, enhance insulin utilization, and even lower the risk of long-term health issues. To increase your diet's polyphenols, select foods like berries, dark chocolate, green tea, red wine, and extra-virgin olive oil. Rich sources include apples, blueberries, cherries, spinach, and kale. Consuming these foods benefits your overall health and helps you manage your weight and control diabetes more effectively by reducing inflammation and improving insulin efficiency.

PRINCIPLE 6: CHOOSE FLAVONOID-RICH FOODS

Flavonoids are a group of antioxidants that are beneficial to your health, especially in the Low GL diabetes diet. Like polyphenols, flavonoids help reduce inflammation and enhance how your body utilizes insulin, which is crucial for preventing chronic diseases. Foods high in flavonoids include berries, apples, onions, and drinks such as green and black teas, red wine, and dark chocolate. Other excellent sources are blueberries, cherries, spinach, and kale. Including these foods in your diet can combat inflammation, improve your body's insulin response, and be advantageous if you aim to lose weight or better manage your diabetes. By focusing on antioxidant-rich foods like polyphenols and flavonoids, you're managing your blood sugar levels and taking steps to protect your brain, potentially reduce your cancer risk, and maintain healthy blood vessels.

PRINCIPLE 7: OPT FOR HEALTHY FATS

The right fats are essential in a healthy low-GL diabetes diet, ensuring your body receives the necessary energy and nutrients for optimal functioning. A well-rounded low-GL diabetes diet should emphasize a balanced intake of fats, mainly monounsaturated and polyunsaturated fats. These fats are vital for good health, providing energy and aiding in absorbing essential vitamins and minerals. Monounsaturated fats in foods benefit heart health by enhancing cholesterol levels, lowering inflammation, and decreasing the risk of heart disease. Polyunsaturated fats in fatty fish and seeds are important for brain function and eye health. As discussed in the previous chapter, "Fats: The Good, The Bad, and The Healthy," there's an ongoing debate about saturated fats, typically found in animal products like meat and dairy. The Dietary Guidelines for Americans advise limiting saturated fat to less than 10% of your daily caloric intake.

PRINCIPLE 8: BOOST OMEGA-3 FATTY ACID INTAKE

The GL diabetes diet emphasizes increasing omega-3 fatty acid consumption and reducing omega-6 fatty acids, contrasting with the typical Western diet where the omega-6/omega-3 ratio has escalated to between 10:1 and 20:1. This imbalance primarily due to modern agricultural practices and agribusiness strategies, has increased reliance on grain-fed animal products and certain vegetable oils like corn, sunflower, safflower, cottonseed, and soybean oils, which are high in omega-6 fats but lack sufficient omega-3s. Omega-6 and omega-3 polyunsaturated fats are essential in various bodily functions, including reproductive, physiological, and immunological processes. Omega-3 fatty acids are crucial in diabetes management as they significantly reduce heart disease risk and support overall health. High levels of omega-6 fats can lead to inflammation and other health complications. Studies have shown that maintaining a balanced omega-6/omega-3 ratio, ideally between 4:1 and 3:1, is key to optimal health, especially for those with diabetes. To increase your omega-3 intake, add omega-3-rich nuts and seeds to your diet. Additionally, fatty fish such as salmon, sardines, anchovies, herring, and mackerel are excellent sources of omega-3s. Regularly including these foods in your meals helps achieve a better omega-3 to omega-6 ratio and provides comprehensive nutritional benefits, making them a crucial part of a diet aimed at diabetes management.

PRINCIPLE 9: ADD ANTI-INFLAMMATORY SPICES TO YOUR DIET

Incorporating anti-inflammatory herbs and spices into your meals is an excellent way to enhance both the flavor and health benefits. Beyond well-known spices like turmeric and garlic, others such as ginger, cinnamon, and cumin also offer anti-inflammatory properties. Integrating fresh herbs into your dishes, using them to replace or reduce salt in recipes, and regularly drinking green tea are additional ways to combat inflammation and boost overall health. While spices and herbs benefit health, they should be seen as complements to, rather than substitutes for, a balanced diet. A healthy Low GL diet should be diverse, including whole grains, fruits, vegetables, lean proteins, and healthy fats. This variety ensures that you're getting a wide range of essential nutrients.

PRINCIPLE 10: AVOID FOODS WITH ARTIFICIAL TRANS FATS

Eliminating artificial trans fats from your low-glycemic load (GL) diet is essential for safeguarding your health and averting the adverse effects associated with these fats. Trans fats are unsaturated fats that naturally occur in small amounts in animal-derived products. However, artificial trans fats, which are industrially produced, pose a significant health risk. Unlike natural trans fats, which are in limited amounts and are not as harmful, artificial trans fats are prevalent in Western diets and have been linked to numerous health issues.

Artificial trans fats are typically found in many processed foods, including fried items like baked goods, frozen pizza, cookies, and crackers, as well as in some margarines and spreads. Among all dietary fats, artificial trans fats are the most harmful. High consumption of these fats is strongly associated with the onset of heart disease and other serious health problems.

These fats are produced through a process known as partial hydrogenation, which turns liquid oils into solid fats like shortening and margarine. Recognizing the dangers of this, the FDA has actively worked to reduce artificial trans fats in the food supply. The health risks of artificial trans fats include:

- Increasing bad cholesterol (LDL).
- Lowering good cholesterol (HDL).
- Raising the risk of cardiovascular disease.
- Contributing to certain types of cancer.
- Exacerbating inflammation.

To effectively limit your daily intake of trans fats, it's essential to read Nutrition Facts labels on packaged foods and inquire about the cooking oils used in restaurants.

PRINCIPLE 11: STAY HYDRATED WITH WATER

Hydration is a fundamental aspect of health. Water regulates body temperature, lubricates joints, and aids in transporting nutrients and removing waste. In the low GL diabetes diet, staying adequately hydrated can also support weight management. Drinking water before meals can induce a sensation of fullness, which may result in decreased food consumption.

Research indicates a link between water consumption and weight loss, although findings are inconclusive. For instance, a study in the journal "Obesity" noted that drinking water before meals correlated with reduced calorie consumption and increased weight loss in overweight and obese participants.

The typical guideline for daily fluid intake is approximately 3 liters (about 13 cups) for men and 2.2 liters (roughly 9 cups) for women. However, these quantities may differ depending on physical activity, environmental conditions, and personal health circumstances.

PRINCIPLE 12: ENGAGE IN REGULAR EXERCISE

Exercise not only aids in weight maintenance and weight loss but also enhances insulin sensitivity, offering significant benefits for regulating blood sugar levels. Moreover, it can decrease the likelihood of developing specific chronic conditions.

Beyond its physical health benefits, regular physical activity positively affects mental health and mood. It can increase energy levels, alleviate stress, improve sleep quality, and boost self-esteem.

Exercise and Blood Sugar Levels:

Moderate Exercise and Hypoglycemia: Moderate-intensity activities like walking or cycling can gradually decrease blood glucose levels. This is because muscles utilize glucose from the bloodstream for energy during prolonged physical activity, effectively lowering blood sugar levels.

High-Intensity Exercise and Hyperglycemia: Conversely, high-intensity exercises such as running or playing vigorous sports can cause an increase in blood glucose levels. This rise is attributed to the body's stress response, which triggers the release of hormones like adrenaline and cortisol. These hormones boost glucose production in the liver and can temporarily decrease insulin sensitivity, resulting in higher blood sugar levels.

Consequently, individuals with diabetes should monitor their blood sugar levels before, during, and after exercising. This monitoring will help understand how different types of physical activities affect their blood glucose and make necessary adjustments to their exercise regimen or diet to maintain optimal blood sugar control.

PRINCIPLE 13: CONSUME NUTS REGULARLY

Nuts are rich in vital vitamins, minerals, and antioxidants. Their calorie density and protein content make them an excellent replacement for other protein sources in your diet, even in small portions. Essential nutrients found in nuts include vitamin E, magnesium, and potassium.

A wealth of epidemiological and clinical research indicates that incorporating nuts into your regular diet can be a valuable strategy for both preventing and managing type 2 diabetes mellitus and related cardiovascular conditions.

PRINCIPLE 14: LIMIT RED MEAT AND ENSURE ADEQUATE PROTEIN

Modifying your diet to include less red meat while maintaining sufficient protein intake aligns well with the principles of the low GL diabetes diet. While red meat is a notable protein source, its consumption has been linked in some studies to an elevated risk of inflammation, chronic diseases, and certain types of cancer. This association is often attributed to high saturated fat and heme iron levels in red meat.

Recent research, however, indicates that unprocessed red meat could be considered safe for individuals with diabetes or prediabetes. This indicates that research findings on red meat and health are mixed, and more studies are necessary for a clearer understanding.

To achieve the health benefits of the low GL diabetes diet, you must moderate red meat consumption and explore alternative protein sources. More detailed guidelines are provided in part IV.

PRINCIPLE 15: EXERCISE CAUTION WITH ALCOHOL CONSUMPTION

The Low GL Diabetes Diet emphasizes the importance of carefully managing alcohol intake for individuals with diabetes. Alcohol, commonly found in social settings, can have a notable effect on blood sugar levels and the overall management of diabetes. The effect of alcohol on glucose metabolism is complex and varies depending on multiple factors, including whether consumed with food or on empty stomach.

In the long term, regular alcohol consumption can pose challenges for diabetes management. For individuals with diabetes who have a balanced diet, alcohol may cause high blood sugar levels. Conversely, those with inadequate dietary intake might experience dangerously low blood sugar levels. Additionally, excessive alcohol intake can lead to the accumulation of harmful acids in the bloodstream and exacerbate various diabetes-related complications, such as disorders of fat metabolism, nerve damage, and eye problems.

Alcohol can also interact with diabetes medications, potentially leading to unpredictable changes in blood sugar levels. Medications such as insulin, sulfonylureas, meglitinides, thiazolidinediones (TZDs), SGLT2 inhibitors, and alpha-glucosidase inhibitors may have altered effects when combined with alcohol.

Furthermore, studies show that HbA1c levels, which reflect long-term blood sugar control, are often higher in individuals with diabetes who consume alcohol compared to non-drinkers.

14
COMMON QUESTIONS & ANSWERS

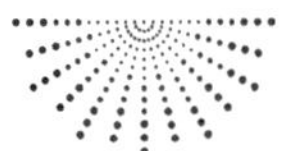

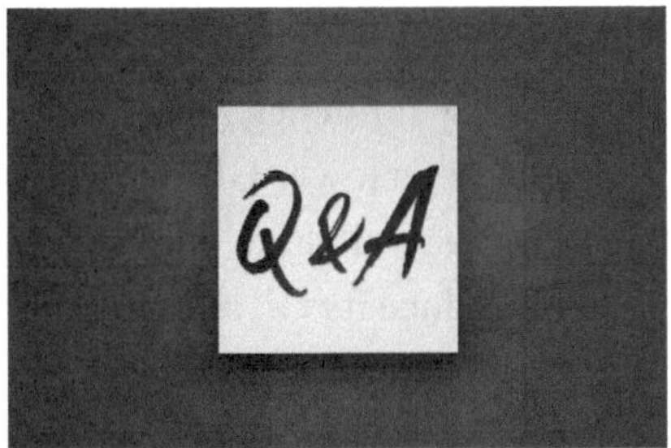

UNDERSTANDING GLYCEMIC INDEX AND GLYCEMIC LOAD

1. **How can the Glycemic Index help in managing diabetes?** The Glycemic Index (GI) significantly aids in diabetes management by guiding individuals to select foods that minimally impact blood glucose levels. Diets low in GI are linked with a substantial reduction in glycated hemoglobin (HbA1c), indicating enhanced control over blood glucose and fewer instances of hypoglycemia. This strategy may reduce the need for medications, lower the likelihood of

complications, and enhance the quality of life for people with diabetes.

2. **What factors influence the Glycemic Index of a food?** The GI of food is affected by several factors, including the type of carbohydrate (simple vs. complex), the method of processing, the cooking technique, and the nutrients composition (e.g., fat and fiber). For instance, whole grains generally have a lower GI than processed grains, and cooking methods with less processing or shorter cooking times tend to yield a lower GI.
3. **How does the ripeness of fruits and vegetables affect their GI and GL?** The ripeness of fruits and vegetables influences their GI and GL because ripening typically increases their sugar content, thereby raising the GI. Opting for less ripe fruits and vegetables is a strategy to lower the overall GI of the diet.
4. **How can cooking methods alter the GI of foods?** Cooking methods can significantly influence the GI of foods. For example, boiling produces a lower GI than baking or frying. Additionally, cooking pasta 'al dente' (slightly firm) rather than entirely soft can reduce its GI, as the firmer texture slows the process of digestion and glucose absorption.
5. **How do food processing methods, such as milling and refining grains, impact the GI?**Food processing methods like milling and refining grains remove bran and germ, lowering the fiber content and increasing the GI. Whole grains digest and absorb more slowly due to their intact fiber, leading to more stable blood glucose levels.
6. **How does the concept of 'al dente' cooking affect the GI of pasta?** Cooking pasta 'al dente' reduces its GI because the firmer texture slows the digestion and absorption of glucose compared to pasta cooked more thoroughly. This cooking method can more effectively manage blood sugar levels after meals.
7. **What is the difference in GI between eating raw fruits and vegetables versus consuming them as juices?** Eating raw

fruits and vegetables typically results in a lower GI than consuming them as juices. Juicing removes fiber, accelerating sugar digestion and absorption, thereby inducing more rapid blood glucose spikes. Whole fruits and vegetables retain fiber, promoting a slower, more incremental increase in blood sugar levels.

8. **Why do some foods have a high GI but a low GL, and how should they be incorporated into a diet?** Foods with a high GI but low GL contain relatively few carbohydrates per serving. These can be balanced with low GI and higher fiber foods within a diet to mitigate the overall impact on blood sugar levels.
9. **How does dehydration or drying fruits and vegetables affect their GL?** Dehydrating or drying fruits and vegetables concentrates their sugars, potentially raising their GL compared to fresh versions. The effect varies based on the dehydration process and the specific fruit or vegetable.
10. **How do sprouting grains or seeds before consuming them affect their GI?** Sprouting grains or seeds changes their nutritional profile, including reducing carbohydrate content and increasing fiber, which can result in a lower GI.
11. **What are Advanced Glycation End-products (AGEs), and how do they relate to the GI of foods?** Advanced Glycation End-products (AGEs) are compounds formed when proteins or fats interact with sugars in the bloodstream. While not directly related to the GI of foods, high-AGE diets can worsen diabetes complications and inflammation. Cooking methods that use lower temperatures and more moisture, such as boiling or steaming, produce fewer AGEs than dry-heat methods like grilling or roasting.
12. **What are the latest research findings on the low GL diet and its impact on diabetes management?** Recent research continues to endorse low GL diets for diabetes management, highlighting glycemic control and insulin sensitivity improvements. Such diets are linked to a reduced risk of type

2 diabetes complications, improved cholesterol levels, and overall health.

NUTRITIONAL STRATEGIES FOR BLOOD SUGAR MANAGEMENT

1. **What are the benefits of following a low GL diabetes diet for someone with diabetes?** A low GL diet offers numerous benefits for individuals with diabetes, including better glycemic control, a reduced risk of hypoglycemic episodes, improved lipid profiles, and a potential decrease in the risk of diabetes-related complications. Additionally, it supports weight management, which is crucial for comprehensive diabetes management.
2. **What strategies can be used to estimate the GI of a food if the value is not available in tables?** To estimate the GI of foods not listed in tables, consider the food's fiber content, degree of processing, and cooking method. Generally, less processed foods, higher in fiber, and cooked in ways that retain their structural integrity (e.g., boiling vs. frying) tend to have a lower GI.
3. **What is the role of fiber in lowering the GL of a meal?** Fiber significantly lowers the GL of a meal by delaying the absorption of carbohydrates, thus slowing sugars release into the bloodstream. This results in a slower, steady rise in blood sugar levels after eating, which helps in enhancing glycemic management.
4. **Q: What are some examples of low GL substitutions for high GL foods?** Low GL substitutions for high GI foods include: • Replacing white bread with whole grain or sourdough bread. • Choosing sweet potatoes over white potatoes. • Choosing whole fruits over fruit juices. • Selecting

legumes and lentils in place of more processed carbohydrate sources, such as white rice.

5. **How can meal timing and frequency impact blood sugar control?** Meal timing and frequency significantly influence blood sugar control. Eating smaller, more frequent meals can stabilize blood glucose levels throughout the day, particularly when these meals are comprised of low-GL foods. This strategy helps mitigate the substantial blood sugar fluctuations often associated with less frequent, larger meals containing high-GL foods.
6. **What is the impact of alcohol and caffeine on blood sugar levels?** Caffeine has been observed to impair blood glucose management in individuals with T2DM, potentially increasing serum insulin, proinsulin, and C-peptide concentrations, indicating an acute caffeine-induced impairment in blood glucose management. Conversely, moderate alcohol consumption appears to have no adverse metabolic effect on blood glucose control and may even lower fasting serum insulin levels in individuals with type 2 diabetes.
7. **How can parents incorporate low GL principles in meals for children with diabetes?** Parents can integrate low GL principles by offering meals and snacks rich in complex carbohydrates with high fiber content, such as whole or minimally-processed grains, legumes, vegetables, and fruits. Incorporating a balance of carbohydrates, protein, and healthy fats can contribute to stabilizing blood sugar levels.

DIETARY COMPONENTS AND THEIR EFFECTS

1. **What is resistant starch, and how does it impact blood sugar levels?** Resistant starch belongs to a category of carbs

that evade digestion in the small intestine and undergo fermentation in the large intestine. Its effect on blood sugar levels is notably lower in comparison to other carbohydrate varieties, as it doesn't prompt a rapid increase in blood glucose levels. Incorporating foods rich in resistant starch into the diet can help prevent post-meal blood sugar spikes.

2. **How does meal fat affect the GI and GL?** The presence of fat in meals can delay gastric emptying, potentially lowering the glycemic response to carbohydrates consumed in the same meal.
3. **What role do protein-rich foods play in a low GL diet?** Protein-rich foods can support a low GL diet by providing satiety and decelerating the digestive process, which helps moderate blood glucose levels. Including protein can also ensure a balanced nutritional profile, resulting in a more steady impact on blood sugar levels.
4. **How do whole grains fit into a low GL diet, and why are they important?** Whole grains are a fundamental component of a low GL diet, typically exhibiting lower GI values than processed grains. They contribute to a slower, more gradual rise in blood glucose levels, partly thanks to their dietary fiber content. This fiber improves digestive health and helps modulate blood glucose responses, making adding a variety of whole grains beneficial for overall health and effective blood sugar management.
5. **How do roasting starches compare to boiling them in terms of affecting their GI?** Roasting starches generally leads to a higher GI compared to boiling. Roasting breaks down starches into simpler sugars that are more readily absorbed, causing quicker blood sugar increases. Boiling maintains more of the food's natural structure, slowing the breakdown of starches into sugars.
6. **How do battering, breading, and frying meats influence the GI and GL of those foods?** Battering, breading, and frying meats can increase the GL due to the addition of

carbohydrates from the batter and bread crumbs, and potentially the GI, as the frying process can alter the structure of carbohydrates. These methods can also raise the meal's calorie content, complicating blood glucose management.

7. **How does consuming dairy products affect the GL of a meal?** Dairy products, especially those high in protein and fat like cheese and yogurt, can lower the GL of a meal by slowing carbohydrate absorption. Fermented dairy products may also have a moderate effect on blood sugar levels.
8. **In what ways can soaking legumes before cooking change their GL?** Soaking legumes before cooking can reduce their GL by lessening antinutrients and sugars that digest slowly, leading to a slower glucose release into the bloodstream.
9. **Q: How do different types of sugars (e.g., fructose vs. glucose) affect the GI of foods?** Different sugars impact the GI differently. Fructose has a lower GI than glucose due to its distinct metabolism, minimally affecting blood sugar levels when consumed in moderation. However, excessive fructose intake, especially from processed foods, can lead to multiple health outcomes, such as insulin resistance, obesity, liver disorders, and diabetes.

PRACTICAL DIETARY MANAGEMENT

1. **How can someone with diabetes effectively incorporate low GL principles when dining out?** When dining out, individuals with diabetes can follow low GL principles by: a.) Choosing dishes with whole grains, legumes, or vegetables are primary ingredients. b.) Requesting dressings and sauces on the side to better control intake. c.) Preferring grilled, baked, or steamed dishes over fried options. d.) Starting with a salad or vegetable-based soup to fill up on lower GL items.

2. **What are the best low-GL snacks for managing hunger between meals?** The best low-GL snacks for managing hunger include: a.) Nuts and seeds. b.) Greek yogurt c.) Fresh fruit. d.) Vegetables with hummus. e.) Whole grain homemade crackers with cheese or nut butter. These snacks deliver a consistent energy source and aid manage hunger between meals.
3. **How can one balance a vegetarian or vegan diet with low GL principles?** Balancing a vegetarian or vegan diet with low GL principles involves selecting plant-based foods that are naturally low in GL, such as whole grains, legumes, nuts, seeds, fruits, and vegetables. Incorporating these foods into your meal planning can assist in stabilizing blood sugar levels while following a vegetarian or vegan dietary regimen.
4. **How does freezing and reheating starchy foods like potatoes or rice affect their GI?** Freezing and then reheating starchy foods can change their structure, potentially lowering their GI by increasing their resistant starch content. This alteration causes the carbohydrates in these foods to digest more slowly, resulting in a slower release of glucose into the bloodstream.
5. **Can adding fats or oils to meals affect the GL, and in what way?** Adding fats or oils to meals can reduce the GL by delaying carbohydrate absorption, thus moderating blood sugar spikes. It's important to select healthy fats and consider the overall calorie content of the meal to maintain a balanced diet.
6. **Can the glycemic response to a meal be moderated by the order in which foods are eaten?** The order of food consumption can influence the glycemic response. Eating proteins and vegetables before carbohydrates can result in a lower glycemic response than consuming carbohydrates first or all meal components together, offering a simple dietary modification to enhance glycemic control.
7. **How do natural sweeteners (e.g., stevia, xylitol) compare to**

sugar in terms of GI?Natural sweeteners like stevia and xylitol have a lower GI than regular sugar. Stevia, a non-nutritive sweetener, has a GI of zero, making it an excellent option for blood sugar control. Xylitol, a sugar alcohol, offers a sweet taste with less impact on the glycemic response.

8. **Can consuming probiotics or fermented foods influence the GL of a meal?** Consuming probiotics or fermented foods may indirectly affect the GL of a meal by improving gut health and glucose metabolism, enhancing the gut microbiota's ability to regulate blood sugar levels.

PART IV
DIETARY GUIDELINES AND MEAL PLANNING PRINCIPLES

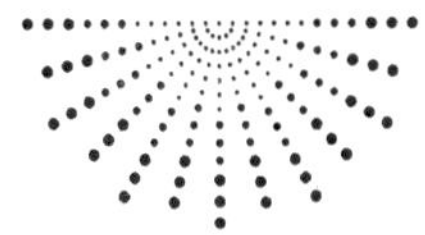

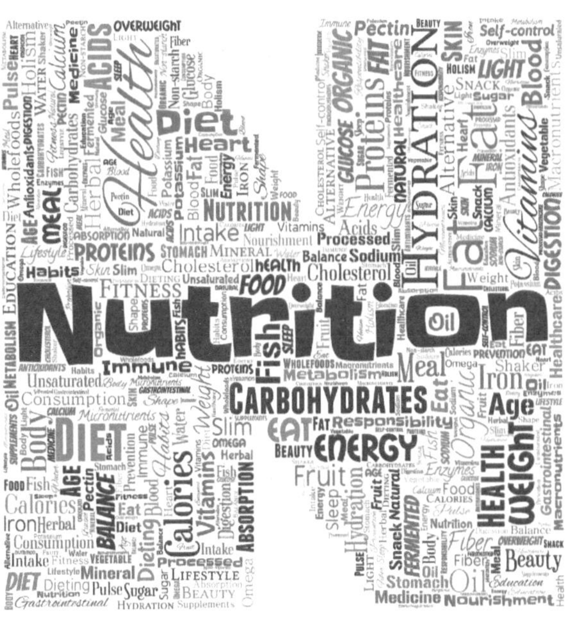

15
MEAL PLANNING GUIDELINES – THE THREE-TIERED APPROACH TO DIABETES MEAL PLANNING

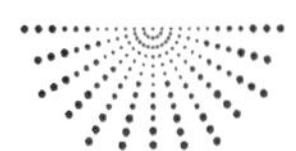

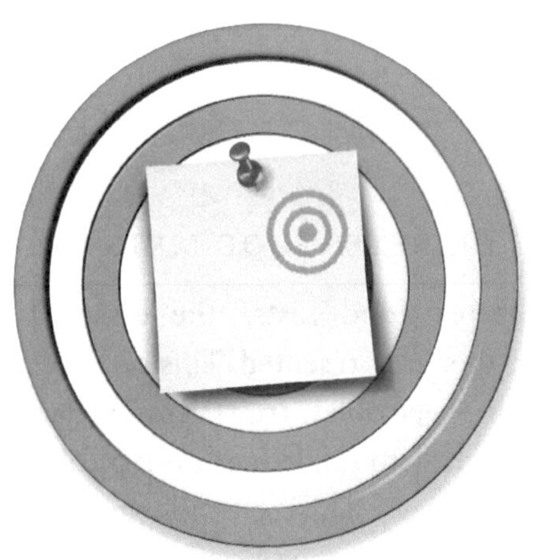

EFFECTIVE DIABETES MEAL PLANNING

Effective diabetes meal planning is a robust process essential for maintaining glycemic control and supporting overall health. This book introduces a structured, three-tiered approach, equipping readers with tools and methods to effectively utilize the glycemic index (GI), glycemic load (GL), and net carb values. This approach progresses from basic to advanced levels.

- **Tier 1: Basic Level - Low GL Diabetes Diet Food Lists:** The initial phase is straightforward and involves Low GL Diabetes Food Lists with comprehensive guidelines to implement the diet effectively.
- **Tier 2: Intermediate Level - The Extensive List with Detailed Nutritional Data**: The second level centers on the Extensive List with Detailed Nutritional Data. This tier is tailored for those prepared to tackle more complex dietary planning, including individuals practicing carbohydrate counting or those on insulin therapy.
- **Tier 3: Advanced Level - Comprehensive Tools**
- The third tier builds on the second, adding a comprehensive GI, GL, and net carb food counter as a complementary tool.

TIER 1: LOW GL DIABETES FOOD LISTS

In "Low GL Diabetes Food Lists," the essentials of initiating a diabetes-conscious diet are presented. This section categorizes fundamental food groups—vegetables, fruits, grains, dairy, and proteins—into clear groups, each with guidelines on typical serving sizes and a brief nutritional overview. This selection goes beyond the basics, adhering to a low GL diet, which is a central theme of this book.

Each food group is labeled as either Low GI and Low GL or Medium GI and Low GL, clearly identifying which foods are optimal for maintaining stable blood sugar levels. This section avoids complex jargon and intricate tables, offering straightforward indicators of which foods fit a low glycemic lifestyle.

This part is designed for ease of use, aiming to mitigate the overwhelm often associated with managing a diabetes diet. It's beneficial when diabetes management becomes daunting, providing a straightforward path back to effective meal planning. Aligned with the 9th Edition of the Dietary Guidelines for Americans and the low GL approach promoted throughout this book, it offers an accessible introduction to incorporating diabetes-friendly foods into daily meals without overwhelming readers with excessive details at once.

TIER 2: THE EXTENSIVE LISTS - DETAILED NUTRITIONAL DATA

These extensive lists form a curated diabetes-friendly food counter, representing the second tier of our three-tiered approach. This methodology has proven effective, leading to optimal outcomes in blood sugar control, preventing complications, and even halting the progression of existing conditions. Recognizing that dietary responses are highly individualized—what works for one may not work for another, even among twins—this advanced tool provides flexibility. You might find Tier 1 sufficient or explore Tiers 2 and 3. The constant goal is to manage your blood sugar level within the therapeutic target and potentially achieve remission. These tools support your journey to better health outcomes, increasing your knowledge and awareness of foods that affect your blood sugar.

Before adding this second approach to this book, we deliberated on the pros and cons for weeks. This approach aligns with universal diabetes recommendations that emphasize tracking total carbohydrates while avoiding simple carbs in favor of complex ones. However, it contrasts with the book's primary approach, which focuses on the physiological impact of foods on blood sugar and the amount of net carbohydrates. We decided to enhance the book with this diabetes-friendly food counter, which is consistent with the Low GL diabetes diet guidelines and specifies serving sizes not exceeding 15 grams of total carbs. This resource eliminates foods with added sugars, unhealthy fats, or those that undergo excessive processing and centers on nutrient-dense, fiber-rich choices.

While this decision may spark discussion, it was made focusing on effectiveness, ease of use, and adherence to international medical recommendations for tracking total carbohydrates, particularly for those on insulin therapy or practicing carbohydrate counting. If you rely on precise carb tracking, the absence of this list will create a gap in this book, forcing you to seek information elsewhere. This food counter remains critically important for those not strictly counting carbs, offering detailed nutritional data on 1,200 foods, with fiber content and serving sizes designed to be at most 15 grams. To facilitate ease of navigation, given the vast amount of information, this resource has been compiled as the second volume of the book, allowing it to be used as a standalone resource.

TIER 3: CONCURRENT USE OF GI, GL, & NET CARB COUNTER AND THE EXTENSIVE LISTS - DETAILED NUTRITIONAL DATA

The GI, GL, & Net Carb Counter represents the culmination of our three-tiered approach, offering the most advanced data on the physiological effects of foods on blood sugar. Its guidelines are straightforward: prioritize foods with a GL under 10, moderate your intake of foods with a GL between 10 and 19 by adjusting serving sizes or frequency, and steer clear of foods with a GL over 20. Your daily intake must be at most 50, aligning with The Centers for Disease Control and Prevention (CDC) recommendations to get at most 10% of your total daily calories from added sugar, which translates to around 50 grams of added sugar.

The evolution of this counter into its current form was notably influenced by direct patient interactions. After distributing a comprehensive 130-page list based on glycemic index research to my patients, I consolidated their feedback and experiences into the 440-page "The Complete Glycemic Index & Glycemic Load Counter for 4000+ Foods" in 2020. This edition, aimed at a broad audience, including those looking to lose weight, manage diabetes or PCOS, or simply follow a GL diet, offered general recommendations. The feedback was invaluable; readers preferred a more refined selection that eliminates ultra-processed foods, sugary beverages, and other items detrimental to blood sugar control, advocating for a focus on healthy, beneficial choices.

Additionally, there was a call for food categorization in alignment with the 9th Edition of Dietary Guidelines for Americans, enhancing usability and adherence to dietary guidelines. As a response, this counter organizes foods into groups, making it easier to find what you're looking for and providing detailed insights into their glycemic effects, net carbohydrates, and recommended serving sizes, all tailored to a glycemic-aware dietary plan.

An entire volume within this book is dedicated to the GI, GL, & Net Carb Counter, following the structured format of Tier 2's Extensive Lists. This volume provides an exhaustive catalog of foods, each detailed by their Glycemic Index, Glycemic Load, and Net Carb content. This comprehensive data allows you to make adequate distinctions between foods based on their potential impact on blood sugar levels.

For example, consider two foods that are both categorized as having a low GL—one with a GL of 2 and another with a GL of 9. While both are in the low GL category, the food with a GL of 9 has an impact on blood sugar that is equivalent to consuming 4.5 times the quantity of the food with a GL of 2. This significant difference highlights the need for nuanced understanding when selecting foods for blood sugar management.

Moreover, understanding the differences between foods with various GI values is equally important. A food with a GI of 20 only raises blood sugar levels to 20% of the response that would be triggered by an equivalent amount of pure glucose. In contrast, a food with a GI of 50 results in a blood sugar rise to 50% of that caused by the same amount of glucose. Recognizing these disparities is vital for managing dietary choices effectively.

16
DIETARY GUIDELINES AND THE STRUCTURED APPROACH OF THE LOW GL DIABETES DIET

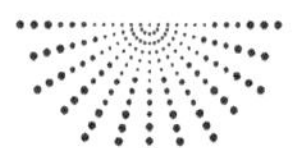

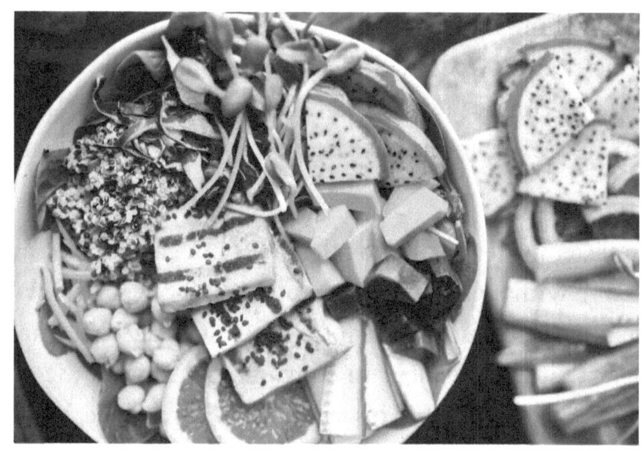

ALIGNMENT WITH CURRENT DIETARY GUIDELINES

The GL Diabetes Diet aligns with the 9th Edition of the Dietary Guidelines for Americans. These guidelines advocate a balanced diet, emphasizing nutrient-dense foods from all food groups while recommending limiting added sugars, saturated fats, and sodium to maintain healthy weight management. The latest Dietary Guidelines provide comprehensive information on recommended dietary practices and are accessible at Dietary Guidelines for Americans 2020-2025 (https://www.dietaryguidelines.gov/sites/default/files/2020-12/Dietary_Guidelines_for_Americans_2020-2025.pdf)

While the 9th Edition of the Dietary Guidelines for Americans does not address diabetes management directly, it offers foundational principles that are highly relevant and adaptable for a diabetes-friendly diet. These guidelines align with the low Glycemic Load (GL) diabetes diet, emphasizing balanced nutrition, moderation, and healthy eating patterns, which are crucial for managing blood sugar levels, promoting heart health, and preventing diabetes-related complications. Here are the guidelines that have been adapted to complement the low GL diabetes diet:

- **Healthy Fats Over Saturated Fats:** Replacing saturated fats with healthy fats found in foods is particularly important for individuals with diabetes, who are at a higher risk of heart disease.
- **Sodium and Blood Pressure Management:** Limiting sodium intake to less than 2,300 milligrams per day, as the guidelines recommend, is crucial for individuals with diabetes to manage blood pressure and reduce the risk of cardiovascular disease.
- **Physical Activity:** Incorporating regular physical activity, as highlighted in the guidelines, is vital for managing diabetes. Physical activity can enhance blood glucose control, lower cardiovascular risk factors, and support weight management.
- **Personalization to Individual Needs:** The guidelines underscore the importance of adapting dietary recommendations to personal preferences, cultural traditions, and specific health needs. For individuals with diabetes, this means tailoring food choices to their dietary requirements, glycemic targets, and other health considerations.
- **Focus on Whole Foods:** Emphasizing whole foods over processed options and supplements can aid in achieving a

more nutrient-dense diet, which is beneficial for managing diabetes and enhancing overall health.

FOOD CATEGORIZATION

Aligned with the classification system from MyPlate.gov, foods are classified into five primary groups:

- Vegetables
- Fruits
- Grains
- Dairy and Fortified Soy Alternatives
- Protein Foods

A sixth category, 'Extras', has been introduced to encompass:

- Beverages
- Dressings and Oils
- Herbs and Spices

Refining Diabetes Management with the Low GL Diabetes Dietary Guidelines

Building on adaptations and categorizations designed to support a comprehensive approach to diabetes management, the Low GL Diabetes Dietary Guidelines enhance this framework by introducing an effective meal planning strategy tailored for those managing diabetes. This includes several key components to help maintain stable blood glucose levels and promote overall health:

1. **Assessment of Nutritional Needs**: Begin by assessing individual caloric needs based on factors like age, sex, weight, activity level, and specific health goals. This assessment helps in customizing the diet plan to ensure it meets the energy requirements without promoting excessive blood sugar

fluctuations.

2. **Adhering to the 15 Core Principles of the Low GL Diabetes Diet**: Embrace the comprehensive set of principles that encapsulate all directives for eating according to the Low GL, Mediterranean Diet, and the 2020-2025 Dietary Guidelines for Americans. These principles provide a holistic framework that covers everything from the types of foods to include in your diet to the appropriate balance of nutrients for optimal health and blood sugar control.
3. **Balanced Meals Across Food Groups**:Structure meals with a balanced combination of carbs, proteins, and fats. This not only aids in nutritional completeness but also ensures a sustained energy release, which helps in keeping stable blood sugar levels throughout the day.
4. **Scheduled Eating Times**: Establish regular meal and snack times to prevent unexpected drops or spikes in blood glucose levels. Consistency in meal timing can significantly enhance metabolic control and reduce the risk of hypoglycemia.
5. **Strategic Snacking**: Plan healthy, strategically timed snacks to manage hunger and prevent overeating during main meals. Choose snacks rich in fiber and protein, such as Greek yogurt with berries or apple slices with almond butter, to maintain satiety and stabilize glucose levels.
6. **Hydration**: Adequate fluid intake is essential, especially for diabetes management, as it facilitates the regulation of blood sugar levels and prevents dehydration. Encourage drinking water and other non-caloric beverages.
7. **Monitoring and Adjustment**: Regular monitoring of blood glucose levels is critical to evaluate the effectiveness of the meal plan. Dietary adjustments should be made based on these readings.
8. **Educational Resources and Support**: Access to reliable resources such as the Diabetes Food Hub, endorsed by the American Diabetes Association (ADA), provides a valuable free tool for finding diabetes-friendly recipes and meal

planning ideas. Additionally, MyPlate.gov offers guidance on portion control and balanced meal planning, aligning with dietary guidelines. Support from dietitians or diabetes educators is also helpful in successfully implementing and adhering to these guidelines. These professionals can provide personalized advice and adjustments to ensure that the diet satisfies dietary needs and fits into the individual's lifestyle.

TYPICAL SERVING SIZE

In the upcoming chapters, detailed guidelines with typical serving sizes will be provided for each food group.

RECIPES

As you'll notice, this book and none of my publications include a cookbook or specific recipes section. Instead, I guide patients and readers to online resources that are not only free but also reliable and effective. I particularly recommend Diabetes Food Hub (https://www.diabetesfoodhub.org/), endorsed by the American Diabetes Association (ADA), as a valuable free tool for finding diabetes-friendly recipes and meal planning ideas.

17
MACRONUTRIENT DISTRIBUTION FOR YOUR LOW GL DIABETES DIET

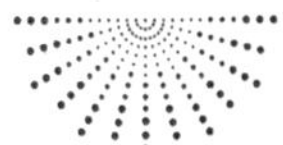

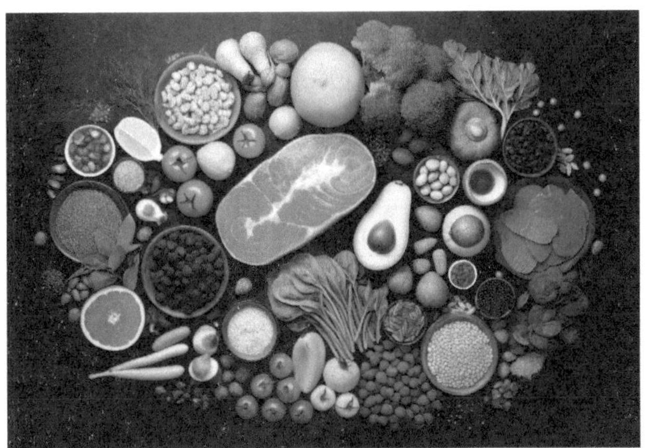

Follow these step-by-step instructions to calculate your macronutrient distribution for a low-GL diabetes Diet comprehensively. These instructions guide you through manual calculations and suggest how online tools can simplify the process.

STEP 1: MEASURE YOUR BASAL METABOLIC RATE (BMR)

Start by calculating your BMR which reflects the number of calories your body needs to perform basic life-sustaining functions like breathing, circulation, and cell production when at rest. (utilizing the Mifflin-St Jeor equation).

For Men:

$$\text{BMR} = 10 \times \text{weight (kg)} + 6.25 \times \text{height (cm)} - 5 \times \text{age (y)} + 5$$

For Women:

$$\text{BMR} = 10 \times \text{weight (kg)} + 6.25 \times \text{height (cm)} - 5 \times \text{age (y)} - 161$$

Alternatively, you can use a reliable online BMR calculator like MyFitnessPal (https://www.myfitnesspal.com/tools/bmr-calculator), which computes these values for you upon entering your weight, height, age, and gender.

Step 2: Determine Total Daily Energy Expenditure (TDEE)

Multiply your BMR by the relevant activity factor to calculate your TDEE. This measurement adjusts for your daily activity and exercise level, providing a more accurate estimate of your total caloric needs.

- Sedentary (little or no exercise): BMR × 1.2
- Lightly active (light exercise/sports 1-3 days/week): BMR × 1.375
- Moderately active (moderate exercise/sports 3-5 days/week): BMR × 1.55
- Very active (hard exercise/sports 6-7 days a week): BMR × 1.725
- Super active (very hard exercise/physical job & exercise 2x a day): BMR × 1.9

Alternatively, Use an online TDEE calculator such as TDEE Calculator (https://tdeecalculator.net/), or **MyFitnessPal** (https://www.myfitnesspal.com/tools/bmr-calculator) to automatically factor in your activity level and provide an estimate.

STEP 3: CALCULATE MACRONUTRIENT DISTRIBUTION

With your TDEE known, allocate your calories among carbohydrates, proteins, and fats. Remember to prioritize the quality of these macronutrients to manage your diabetes effectively.

Carbohydrates: Aim for 45-50% of your total calories. Choose high-quality carbohydrates that have a low glycemic load.

Proteins: Your protein needs can vary:

- Normal weight without CKD: 0.8 to 1.2 grams per kg body weight.
- Overweight or obese: 1.5 to 2 grams per kg body weight.
- With early-stage CKD: 0.8 to 1 gram per kg body weight.
- Advanced CKD: 0.6 to 0.8 grams per kg body weight.

Fats: Allocate the remaining calories to fats, focusing on sources rich in monounsaturated and polyunsaturated fats.

STEP 4: CONVERT MACRONUTRIENT PERCENTAGES INTO GRAMS

To translate the calorie percentages into grams:

- Carbohydrates and proteins provide 4 calories per gram.
- Fats provide 9 calories per gram.

For a 2000-calorie diet:

- **Carbohydrates:** 50% of 2000 calories = 1000 calories → $\frac{1000 \text{ calories}}{4 \text{ cal/g}} = 250 \text{ grams}$
- **Proteins:** 20% of 2000 calories = 400 calories → $\frac{400 \text{ calories}}{4 \text{ cal/g}} = 100 \text{ grams}$
- **Fats:** 30% of 2000 calories = 600 calories → $\frac{600 \text{ calories}}{9 \text{ cal/g}} = 67 \text{ grams}$

STEP 5: CONTINUOUSLY MONITOR AND ADJUST

Regularly monitor your health and adjust your macronutrient intake as needed. This helps manage your diabetes more effectively and aligns with your health goals. Pay particular attention to how your body responds to different macronutrient distributions and adjust based on your metabolic health, blood sugar responses, and overall well-being.

By following these detailed steps, you can tailor your diet to manage diabetes through a controlled and informed approach to macronutrient distribution. Whether you calculate manually or use online tools, the key is consistency and regular adjustment based on real-world outcomes.

18
THE PLATE METHOD

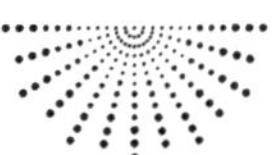

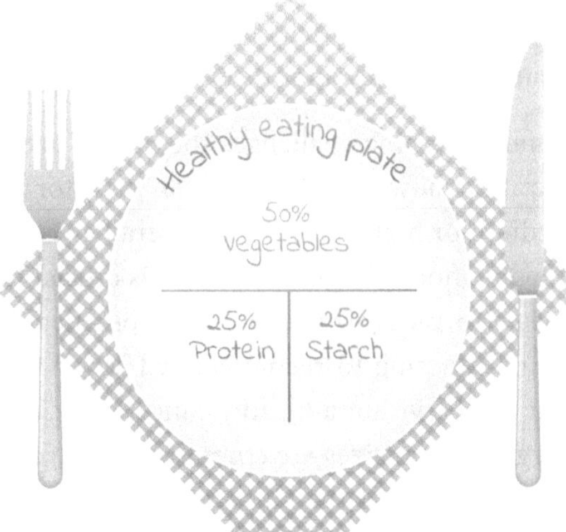

THE IMPORTANCE OF PORTION CONTROL

Understanding portion control is crucial for managing a diabetes diet, particularly when considering the Glycemic Load of foods. A critical aspect to grasp is that even foods categorized as having a low GL can lead to increased glycemic responses if consumed in quantities larger than the standard serving size. This is because GL values are directly influenced by portion size; consuming more than the typical serving can elevate the GL of a meal, thereby increasing the amount of glucose entering the bloodstream, similar to consuming pure glucose.

For instance, a food item with a low GL may be perceived as a healthier choice for managing blood sugar levels. However, if one consumes a double portion of this food, the ingested GL—and consequently, its physiological impact—could escalate to a range considered medium or even high. This shift underscores that each unit of GL is equivalent to the effect of consuming 1 gram of pure glucose. Therefore, while a food may initially be classified as low GL, excessive consumption can substantially alter its glycemic impact.

This nuanced understanding challenges the notion of static GL categories by illustrating how portion size can transform a food's GL from low to medium or high, affecting its overall glycemic impact. It's a concept that, while not universally applied, is crucial for individuals managing diabetes to recognize. The goal is practical: to emphasize the importance of adhering to recommended serving sizes to maintain blood sugar levels within a healthy range, especially in environments where large portion sizes are common. This approach fosters a more accurate application of the GL system, enabling individuals to make informed choices about their diet.

THE PLATE METHOD: SIMPLIFYING DIETARY MANAGEMENT

In the last chapter, we explored the technique of calculating macronutrient distribution, an advanced technique for customizing meals in the low GL diabetes diet. Though initially daunting, this approach is incredibly effective for enhancing diet adherence and fine-tuning food intake, tailored explicitly for diabetes management. It allows for high personalization, ensuring that eating habits align perfectly with an individual's energy needs, health status, and personal preferences, thereby improving blood sugar control and nutritional health.

For beginners, a more straightforward method focuses on adjusting daily food portions to positively impact glycemic load and overall diet management without the complexity of tracking every macronutrient. This approach makes it easier to manage diets effectively and offers a good starting point for those looking to understand and control their dietary intake.

THE PLATE METHOD EXPLAINED

- **Vegetables:** Fill half your plate with colorful, non-starchy vegetables
- **Protein:** Use one quarter of your plate for lean protein sources
- **Carbohydrates:** The remaining quarter is for carbohydrate-rich foods

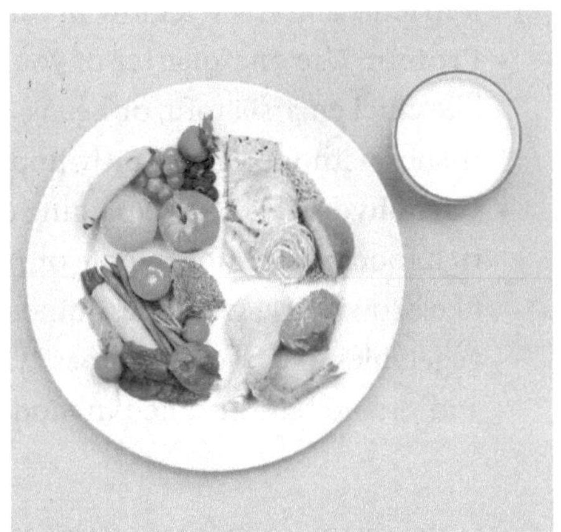

The Plate Method is an intuitive, visually based strategy for assembling meals that naturally regulate portion size and nutrient balance. Here's how it works:

- **Divide your plate into sections**: Half is filled with non-starchy vegetables, one quarter with lean protein, and the remaining quarter with whole, minimally processed grains or starchy vegetables. This distribution helps control portions while ensuring a balanced intake of nutrients.

- **Choose your foods wisely**: Focus on incorporating a variety of colors and kinds of vegetables to maximize nutrient intake. Select lean proteins to support muscle health without excessive fat intake. Opt for whole grains or starchy vegetables to get enough fiber and energy.

IMPLEMENTING THE PLATE METHOD

Start with a standard 9-inch dinner plate to prevent overeating by restricting the quantity of food that can fit on the plate.

- **Vegetables**: Fill half your plate with colorful, non-starchy vegetables (e.g. leafy greens, peppers, broccoli), rich in nutrients and fiber yet low in calories and carbohydrates.
- **Protein**: Use one-quarter of your plate for protein sources like chicken, fish, tofu, or beans, which help build and repair tissues without significantly impacting blood sugar levels.
- **Carbohydrates**: The remaining quarter is for carbohydrate-rich foods, preferably whole or minimally processed grains like brown rice, wild rice, quinoa, buckwheat or starchy vegetables like sweet potatoes. These provide essential energy and should be consumed in moderation.

ADVANTAGES AND LIMITATIONS OF THE PLATE METHOD

The Plate Method offers simplicity and flexibility and promotes balanced eating, automatically ensuring a balanced intake of macronutrients and aiding in weight management and glycemic control. However, for those who require strict blood sugar management or have additional health issues like chronic kidney disease, the method might not offer the detailed guidance necessary for effective condition management. Although it provides an essential structure for healthy eating, it may not fully address the unique dietary needs stemming from specific health conditions, levels of physical activity, or dietary restrictions.

Nevertheless, the Plate Method remains a practical and visually engaging strategy for diet management, particularly appealing to those who prefer a straightforward approach to

Nevertheless, the Plate Method remains a practical and visually engaging strategy for diet management, particularly appealing to those who prefer a straightforward approach to healthy eating. While it may not meet the need for precise customization in every case, it establishes a strong foundation for beginning the low GL diabetes diet, which is especially beneficial for newcomers to dietary management.

19
CRAFTING A ONE-DAY MEAL PLAN

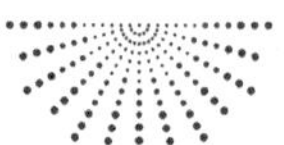

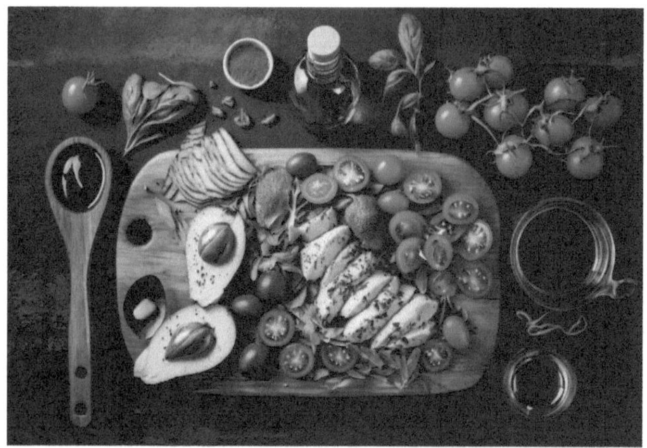

This chapter offers an extensive guide on how to design daily or weekly meal plans that adhere to the principles of the low GL diabetes diet. Instead of just providing a preset 7-day or 4-week meal plan, it equips you with the necessary skills to create your own meal plans. This approach ensures you understand the reasoning behind each choice, enabling you to become autonomous and proficient in managing your diet effectively.

I. DETAILED ONE-DAY MEAL PLAN WITH SERVING SIZES AND NUTRITIONAL INFORMATION

Objective: Designing your own meal plans is crucial for managing diabetes effectively. It enables you to tailor your diet to your preferences, budget, seasonal availability, and specific health requirements like food intolerances. This structured low glycemic load diabetes diet meal plan is designed for straightforward application, allowing you to adapt it as part of your daily routine rather than sticking to a rigid format.

KEY BENEFITS OF THE STRUCTURED MEAL PLAN:

- **Carbohydrate Management:** Targets 45-50% of daily calories from carbohydrates to aid maintain stable blood sugar levels.
- **Protein Intake:** Ensures optimal daily protein intake, with detailed guidance in the chapter "Protein — The Building Blocks of Life."
- **Healthy Fats:** Balances the remaining calories with healthy fats, as detailed in the chapter "Lipids — Essential Macronutrients for Health."

PLAN COMPLIANCE FEATURES:

- **Low-GL Foods:** Each meal incorporates primarily low-GL foods or ingredients to promote a stable glycemic response.
- **Safe Cooking Methods:** Emphasizes cooking techniques that reduce the formation of advanced glycation end-products (AGEs) and do not increase the glycemic load, such as boiling, roasting, steaming, and poaching. These methods align with dietary guidelines restricting AGEs while maintaining a low GL.

- **Adherence to Core Principles:** Follows 15 core principles to effectively manage a low GL diet.

Although managing your diet with this plan may initially seem daunting, it becomes straightforward with practice. By following the detailed step-by-step guide in the last section, you can ensure consistent application and gradually integrate these practices into your lifestyle, enhancing your health and ability to manage diabetes.

Meal Breakdown: To meet the CDC recommendations of having 45-50% of daily calories come from carbohydrates in a 2000-calorie diet, we need to adjust the meal plan to include 225 grams of total carbohydrates per day. This adjustment also emphasizes the inclusion of fiber-rich foods (20 to 35 grams of fiber daily) to enhance glycemic control and overall health benefits.

BELOW IS THE MEAL PLAN:

Total Daily Carbohydrates: Approximately 225 grams, including 20 to 35 grams of fiber. 225 grams equates to 900 calories because each gram is 4 calories. On a 2000-calorie diet, this ensures that 45% of daily calories come from carbohydrates.

Breakfast:

- **Dish:** Oatmeal with Berries, Almonds, and Chia Seeds
- **Serving Size:** ¾ cup cooked oatmeal, 1 cup fresh berries, 10 almonds, 1 tablespoon chia seeds
- **Carbohydrates:** Approx. 50 grams
- **Description:** Oats provide a slow-releasing carbohydrate source. Berries add fiber, almonds contribute healthy fats and protein, and chia seeds increase the fiber content, making for a nutrient-dense start to the day.

Morning Snack:

- **Dish:** Greek Yogurt with Raspberries and a Drizzle of Honey
- **Serving Size:** 1 cup Greek yogurt, 1 cup raspberries, 1 teaspoon honey
- **Carbohydrates:** Approx. 30 grams
- **Description:** Greek yogurt is high in protein, raspberries are rich in fiber, and a small amount of honey provides a natural sweetener without significantly impacting the glycemic load.

Lunch:

- **Dish:** Quinoa Salad with Mixed Greens, Cherry Tomatoes, Grilled Chicken, Avocado, and Vinaigrette
- **Serving Size:** 1 cup cooked quinoa, 2 cups mixed greens, ½ cup cherry tomatoes, 4 oz grilled chicken, ½ sliced avocado, 2 tablespoons vinaigrette
- **Carbohydrates:** Approx. 50 grams
- **Description:** Quinoa and mixed greens serve as low GI carbohydrate sources, chicken provides protein, avocado offers healthy fats, and tomatoes add additional fiber and nutrients.

Afternoon Snack:

- **Dish:** Whole Wheat Pita with Hummus and Sliced Cucumber
- **Serving Size:** 1 small whole wheat pita, 3 tablespoons hummus, ½ cup sliced cucumber
- **Carbohydrates:** Approx. 30 grams
- **Description:** Whole wheat pita provides complex carbohydrates and fiber, hummus contributes protein and fat, and cucumber offers hydration and additional nutrients.

Dinner:

- **Dish:** Grilled Salmon with Sweet Potato and Steamed Broccoli
- **Serving Size:** 5 oz grilled salmon, 1 medium sweet potato, 1 cup steamed broccoli
- **Carbohydrates:** Approx. 45 grams
- **Description:** Salmon is rich in omega-3 fatty acids, sweet potato is a high-fiber carbohydrate source, and broccoli is packed with nutrients and fiber for a balanced meal.

Evening Snack:

- **Dish:** Pear with a Slice of Cheese
- **Serving Size:** 1 medium pear, 1 slice of cheese
- **Carbohydrates:** Approx. 20 grams
- **Description:** Pear provides a low GI, fiber-rich fruit option, paired with cheese for protein and fat, rounding out the day with a balanced snack.

II. STEP-BY-STEP GUIDE TO CRAFTING A DIABETES-FRIENDLY MEAL PLAN

This section outlines a structured approach to crafting daily meal plans in accordance with the three-tiered structure of the GL Diabetes Diet. It aims to ensure that these plans cater to the diverse needs of individuals at diverse stages of dietary management. This guide emphasizes the importance of developing personalized meal plans tailored to specific nutritional requirements and management objectives.

STEP 1: SELECT APPROPRIATE FOOD LISTS BASED ON YOUR TIER

- **Tier 1 Adopters:** Use the Diabetes-Friendly Food List for Tier 1, focusing on low GL foods that do not require carb counting. This is ideal for those new to diabetes management.
- **Tier 2 Adopters:** Refer to the Extensive List with Nutritional Data for precise carbohydrate tracking, suitable for those managing diabetes with insulin therapy.
- **Tier 3 Adopters:** Utilize resources that include detailed GI, GL, and Net Carb data for meticulous dietary control required to manage complex diabetes conditions.

STEP 2: CALCULATE DAILY CALORIC NEED

- Determine your daily caloric requirements using tools such as an online TDEE calculator like TDEE Calculator (https://tdeecalculator.net/), or MyFitnessPal (https://www.myfitnesspal.com/tools/bmr-calculator). These resources provide personalized estimates of needed calories, carbs, fat, protein, and BMI, helping you tailor your meal plan to your specific health requirements and lifestyle.

STEP 3: PLAN MACRONUTRIENT DISTRIBUTION

- **45-50% Carbohydrates:** Following the dietary guidelines, ensure that 45-50% of your daily caloric intake comes from carbohydrates. Alternatively, use the Plate Method to visually divide your plate into sections—half of it filled with non-starchy vegetables, one-quarter with protein sources, and one-quarter with whole grains or starchy vegetables.

STEP 4: ADHERE TO RECOMMENDED SERVING SIZES

- Ensure that the serving sizes comply with those provided in the relevant lists. This consistency helps achieve the desired balance of nutrients without exceeding carbohydrate limits that could impact glycemic control.

STEP 5: UTILIZE THE 15 CORE PRINCIPLES CHECKLIST

- Develop a checklist incorporating all 15 core principles, ensuring that each meal and snack aligns with these guidelines for a comprehensive approach to diabetes management. Examples of actions include checking for low-glycemic index foods, increasing olive oil consumption, and ensuring adequate hydration.

15 core principles Checklist

STEP	TASK	DONE
01	Check for Low-Glycemic Index Foods in each meal	
02	Increase Olive Oil Consumption in your cooking.	
03	Limit Added Sugar Intake throughout the day.	
04	Reduce Sodium Intake by choosing low-salt options.	
05	Include Polyphenol-Rich Foods in your diet.	
06	Select Flavonoid-Rich Foods when choosing fruits and vegetables.	
07	Use Healthy Fats in meal preparations.	
08	Ensure Omega-3 Fatty Acids are present in your meals.	
09	Add Anti-Inflammatory Spices to enhance flavors naturally.	
10	Avoid Foods with Artificial Trans Fats entirely.	
11	Drink plenty of water to maintain hydration.	
12	Plan for Regular Physical Activity each day.	
13	Incorporate Regular Nut Consumption into snacks or meals.	
14	Control Red Meat Intake but ensure adequate protein	
15	Monitor Alcohol Consumption, keeping it minimal and occasional.	

STEP 6: CHOOSE COMPLIANT COOKING METHODS AND TIMES

- Opt for cooking methods that do not increase the glycemic load, such as steaming, boiling, and poaching. Avoid methods that raise the glycemic index, like frying and excessive roasting.
- Monitor cooking times to prevent overcooking, especially for carbohydrates affecting their GI.

IMPLEMENTATION TIPS:

- **Plan Ahead:** Allocate weekly time to plan your meals according to these guidelines.
- **Cook in Batches:** Prepare meals in batches to save time and ensure consistency in serving sizes and cooking methods.
- **Regular Reviews:** Periodically review your meal plan against your health outcomes and adjust as necessary in consultation with a dietitian.

By following these structured steps, you can create effective meal plans that meet your dietary needs and integrate seamlessly into a healthy lifestyle. This guide ensures that all aspects of meal planning, from caloric intake to cooking methods, are designed to sustain stable blood sugar levels and promote overall well-being.

PART V
LOW GL DIABETES DIET FOOD LISTS

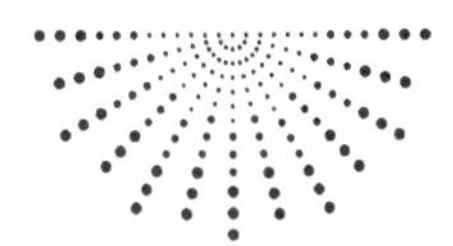

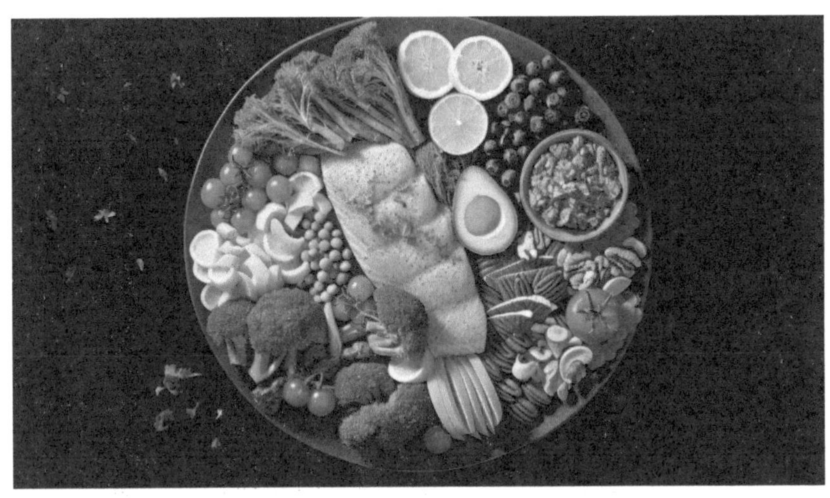

20

THE VEGETABLES DIABETES-FRIENDLY FOOD LISTS

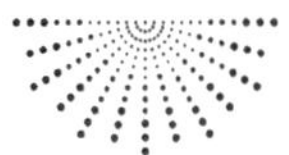

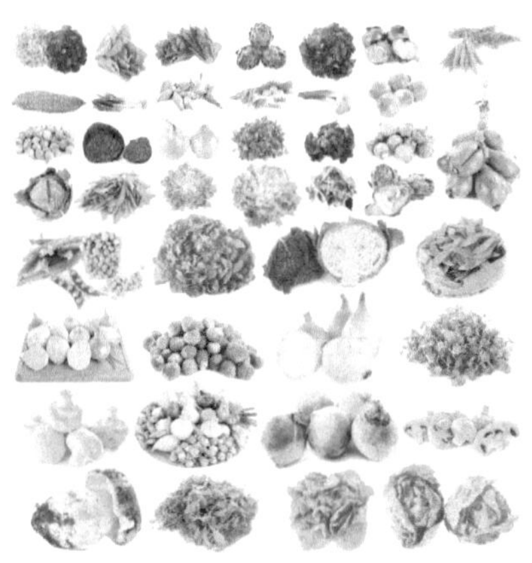

The low glycemic load diabetes diet strongly emphasizes a consistent and diverse intake of vegetables due to their nutrient-dense composition. Vegetables are particularly noteworthy for their high concentrations of dietary fiber, vitamins, minerals, and an array of beneficial phytochemicals, including polyphenols, flavonoids, beta-carotene, anthocyanidins, and carotenoids. Notably, research by Darmon et al. (2005) highlights that fruits and vegetables achieve high nutrient density scores primarily because they are nutrient-rich relative to their low energy content. They also offer a favorable nutrient-to-price ratio, providing vital nutrients at a reasonable cost compared to other food groups.

According to MyPlate.gov, vegetables are categorized into five subgroups, each defined by its distinctive nutrient contributions:

1. **Dark-green vegetables:** These foods are abundant in essential nutrients, including vitamins A, C, E, and K, and minerals like iron, calcium, and potassium. Their potent antioxidant properties contribute to the prevention of chronic illnesses, including various cancers and heart diseases.
2. **Red & Orange Vegetables:** These vegetables are abundant in vitamins A and C and are celebrated for their potent antioxidant properties, which are instrumental in disease prevention.
3. **Legumes (Beans, Peas, Lentils):** As excellent sources of plant-based protein and fiber, legumes have a low glycemic index, which is beneficial for stable blood sugar management, making them essential for those with diabetes.
4. **Starchy Vegetables:** Although these vegetables are higher in carbohydrates, they remain a crucial part of a balanced diet by providing essential nutrients. For individuals with diabetes, careful portion control is necessary.
5. **Other Vegetables:** This category encompasses various vegetables, each with a unique nutritional profile. They are typically lower in carbohydrates than their starchy counterparts and rich in vitamins and minerals.

STARCHY VS NON-STARCHY VEGETABLES

The primary distinction between starchy and non-starchy vegetables in the context of the low GL diabetes diet lies in their carbohydrate content, how this affects blood sugar levels, and their role in weight management. Starchy vegetables such as potatoes, corn, peas, plantains, yams, carrots, sweet potatoes, and parsnips have a higher carbohydrate and calorie content than non-starchy vegetables. While they contain starch, a complex carbohydrate broken down into glucose by the body, it's not the sole factor influencing blood sugar levels. However, starchy vegetables tend to have a higher GL due to their higher carbohydrate content, so careful portion control is essential in the low GL diet.

NUTRITIONAL PROFILE:

Starchy Vegetables:

- **Higher in Calories:** More calories per serving due to higher carbohydrate content.
- **Carbohydrates:** Good source of complex carbohydrates, offering a steady release of energy.
- **Fiber:** Often rich in fiber, especially in their skins.
- **Vitamins and Minerals:** High in vitamin C, potassium, and vitamin B6.
- **Higher Energy Density:** Their higher carbohydrate content means they provide more energy per unit weight, contributing to a higher GL.

Non-Starchy Vegetables:

- **Lower in Calories:** Fewer calories and carbohydrates.
- **Carbohydrates:** Contain less starch and more fiber, which does not raise blood sugar significantly.
- **Fiber:** High fiber content supports digestive health and helps maintain satiety for longer periods.
- **Vitamins and Minerals:** Abundant in vitamins A, C, and K, and antioxidants. Leafy greens are also rich in iron and calcium.

- **Lower in Energy Density:** Less dense in calories and carbohydrates per unit weight, making them favorable for weight management.

Density Differences:

- **Starchy Vegetables:** Tend to be heartier and provide a denser mouthfeel, which can be more satisfying in meals.
- **Non-Starchy Vegetables:** More water-rich, contributing to a less dense texture, ideal for calorie control and weight management.

Incorporating non-starchy vegetables into the diet is particularly beneficial for managing type 2 diabetes mellitus (T2DM) as per the twin cycle hypothesis, which posits that weight loss is crucial for reversing the cycle of insulin resistance and beta-cell dysfunction typical in T2DM. Non-starchy vegetables, with their lower GL and caloric content, play a significant role in dietary strategies aimed at weight loss and optimal blood sugar management. This approach aligns with the principles of the low GL diabetes diet, which prioritizes foods that have minimal impact on glycemic variability, supporting overall diabetes management and contributing to long-term health improvements.

Extensive research consistently demonstrates that a diet abundant in fruits and vegetables is not just good for your overall health, but also linked to a decreased likelihood of developing type 2 diabetes-related complications. This protective effect is primarily due to their antioxidant content, fiber, and nutrient density.

BEANS, PEAS, LENTILS

The food group consisting of beans, peas, and lentils is highly beneficial for individuals following a low glycemic load (GL) diabetes diet.

Why Include Beans, Peas, and Lentils in the Low GL Diabetes Diet?

- **Low Glycemic Index**: Most beans, peas, and lentils have a low GI, meaning lead to a more gradual and reduced increase in blood sugar levels following meals.
- **High Fiber Content**: The abundant fiber slows down the absorption of glucose and improves overall digestive health.
- **Rich in Protein**: Protein is crucial for blood sugar management because it can enhance satiety and help avoid sharp increases in glucose levels after meals.
- **Nutrient Dense**: These foods are packed with essential vitamins and minerals, including potassium, iron, magnesium, phosphorus and B vitamins, supporting overall health beyond just diabetes management.

PORTION SIZES AND INTAKE RECOMMENDATIONS

Adhering to dietary guidelines that promote stable blood sugar levels is critical for adequate diabetes management. This means understanding the right serving sizes for vegetables, especially their carbohydrate content. Ideally, each serving should not exceed 15 grams of carbohydrates. However, it's concerning that most Americans fail to consume the advised daily intake of fruits and vegetables. This shortfall can significantly impact overall health and diabetes management, underscoring the importance of meeting these recommendations.

Guidelines for Vegetable Intake for Diabetes Management:

- **Carbohydrate Management**: Each serving of vegetables is limited to containing about 15 grams of carbohydrates to comply with authoritative organizations' guidelines.

- **Daily Recommendations**: Adults should generally consume at least 2-3 cups of vegetables per day as part of a balanced diet.

Here's a table summarizing the serving sizes for different vegetable subgroups, each designed to contain no more than 15 grams of carbohydrates and the general daily recommendation:

Vegetable Subgroup	Serving Size	Carbohydrate Content (Approx.)	Daily Recommended Servings
Dark-Green Vegetables	1 cup (cooked or raw)	<5 grams	1-2 servings
Red and Orange Vegetables	1/2 cup (cooked)	15 grams	1-2 servings
Starchy Vegetables	1/2 cup (cooked)	15 grams	1 serving
Beans and Peas (Legumes)	1/3 cup (cooked)	15 grams	1 serving
Other Vegetables	1 cup (raw or cooked)	<5 grams	1-2 servings

THE LOW-GL DIABETES FOOD LISTS

Dark-Green Vegetables

- **Amaranth Leaves (all forms)** — Low GI, low GL. Rich in vitamins A, C, and folate, and a good source of dietary fiber which helps in blood sugar regulation.
- **Arugula (Rocket) (all forms)** — Low GI, negligible GL. High in calcium, potassium, folate, and vitamin K, beneficial for maintaining stable blood glucose levels.
- **Asparagus (all forms)** — Low GI, low GL. Offers a good source of fiber, vitamins A, C, E, and K, and is particularly high in folate.

- **Beet Greens (all forms)** — Low GI, low GL. High in fiber, vitamin A, vitamin C, and potassium, aiding in glycemic control and overall health.
- **Bok Choy (Chinese Chard) (all forms)** — Low GI, very low GL. Contains high levels of vitamins A, C, and K, and is rich in calcium and iron.
- **Broccoli (all forms)** — Low GI, very low GL. Excellent source of dietary fiber, vitamins C and K, and contains bioactive compounds that may assist in reducing blood sugar levels.
- **Brussels Sprouts (all forms)** — Low GI, low GL. High in fiber, vitamins C and K, and numerous nutrients that support metabolic health.
- **Chamnamul (all forms)** — Low GI, low GL. Typically high in vitamins and minerals, aids in digestion and has antioxidant properties.
- **Chard (all forms)** — Low GI, low GL. Great source of vitamins A, C, and K, magnesium, manganese, iron, and dietary fiber.
- **Collards (all forms)** — Low GI, low GL. Rich in vitamins A, C, and K, and fiber, which helps to stabilize blood sugar.
- **Dandelion Greens (all forms)** — Low GI, low GL. Packed with calcium, iron, fiber, and vitamins A and K, which are beneficial for blood sugar management.
- **Endive (all forms)** — Low GI, very low GL. High in fiber and vitamins A and K, with a minimal impact on blood sugar.
- **Kale (all forms)** — Low GI, low GL. Very high in vitamins A, C, K, and significant amounts of minerals and antioxidants.
- **Kohlrabi Greens (all forms)** — Low GI, low GL. Contains fiber, vitamins A, C, and K, contributing to low glycemic responses.
- **Mesclun Greens (typically raw)** — Low GI, negligible GL. A mix that usually includes a variety of nutrient-rich, low GI leafy greens.
- **Mustard Greens (all forms)** — Low GI, low GL. Provides a rich source of fiber, vitamins A, C, and K, and antioxidants.

- **Nasturtium Leaves (typically raw)** — Low GI, negligible GL. Known for their high vitamin C content and unique peppery flavor.
- **Poke Greens (all forms)** — Low GI, low GL. Must be cooked properly to neutralize toxins; high in vitamins A and C once safely prepared.
- **Rapini (Broccoli Raab) (all forms)** — Low GI, low GL. High in vitamins A, C, and K, and includes beneficial plant compounds that may help manage blood sugar.
- **Romaine Lettuce (all forms)** — Very low GI, negligible GL. High in fiber, vitamins A, C, K, and folate.
- **Sorrel (all forms)** — Low GI, low GL. Rich in vitamins A and C, beneficial for blood sugar control due to its high content of dietary fiber.
- **Spinach (all forms)** — Low GI, low GL. Extremely high in vitamin K, and good amounts of manganese, folate, and iron.
- **Swiss Chard (all forms)** — Low GI, low GL. Excellent source of fiber, vitamins A, C, and K, magnesium, and potassium.
- **Taro Leaves (all forms)** — Low GI, low GL when cooked. High in vitamins A and C, fiber, and several other essential nutrients.
- **Turnip Greens (all forms)** — Low GI, low GL. High in calcium, folate, fiber, and vitamins A, C, and K.
- **Watercress (all forms)** — Very low GI, negligible GL. High in vitamins A, C, and K, and provides potent antioxidant benefits.

Red and Orange Vegetables

- **Acorn Squash (all forms)** — Moderate GI, low GL when consumed in small portions. Rich in vitamins A and C, and a good source of dietary fiber which helps manage blood sugar levels.

- **Beets (all forms)** — Medium GI, low to moderate GL. High in fiber, folate, and manganese, making them beneficial for blood sugar control when eaten in moderation.
- **Butternut Squash (all forms)** — Moderate GI, low GL in controlled portions. Provides significant amounts of vitamins A and C, and is a good source of fiber, aiding in glycemic control.
- **Calabaza (all forms)** — Moderate GI, low GL when portion-controlled. High in vitamin A and C, and provides fiber which assists in maintaining stable blood sugar levels.
- **Carrots (all forms)** — Low to moderate GI, very low GL. High in beta-carotene and fiber, making them ideal for steady blood sugar management and overall health.
- **Chili Peppers (all forms)** — Low GI, negligible GL. Rich in vitamins C and B6, capsaicin, and antioxidants, they contribute minimal sugar impact while enhancing metabolic health.
- **Hubbard Squash (all forms)** — Moderate GI, low GL in controlled portions. Rich in vitamin C and dietary fiber, which aid in maintaining stable blood sugar levels.
- **Orange Bell Peppers (all forms)** — Low GI, very low GL. Excellent sources of vitamins A and C, and fiber, which help in regulating glucose levels and improving insulin sensitivity.
- **Orange Cauliflower (all forms)** — Low GI, very low GL. Offers slightly higher beta-carotene than white varieties, along with high vitamin C and fiber content, beneficial for glycemic control.
- **Paprika (from dried red peppers)** — Low GI, minimal GL. Rich in antioxidants, vitamins A and E, and capsaicin, enhancing flavor without raising blood sugar.
- **Peppadew Peppers (all forms)** — Moderate GI, low GL if unsweetened. They are a good source of vitamin C and dietary fiber, which can assist in moderating blood sugar spikes.
- **Persimmons (typically raw)** — Moderate GI, moderate GL.

They provide good amounts of fiber and vitamins, especially vitamin A and C, but should be eaten cautiously due to natural sugars.

- **Pumpkin (all forms)** — Low GI, low GL. High in fiber and beta-carotene, which the body converts into vitamin A, supporting blood sugar regulation and providing antioxidant benefits.
- **Radishes (typically raw)** — Very low GI, negligible GL. High in vitamin C and other minerals, with very low carbohydrate content, making them an excellent choice for snacks.
- **Red and Orange Bell Peppers (all forms)** — Low GI, very low GL. High in vitamins A and C, with a high nutrient density and fiber, supporting low blood sugar impacts.
- **Red Bell Peppers (all forms)** — Low GI, very low GL. They are exceptionally high in vitamin C, contain a good amount of fiber, and are rich in antioxidants, all of which contribute to effective blood sugar management.
- **Red Cabbage (all forms)** — Low GI, very low GL. Offers a high concentration of vitamins C and K, fiber, and anthocyanins, aiding in both glycemic control and antioxidant protection.
- **Red Kuri Squash (all forms)** — Moderate GI, low GL in small servings. Provides beta-carotene, vitamins C and E, and fiber, helpful for maintaining stable blood glucose levels.
- **Red Onions (all forms)** — Low GI, low GL. Contains quercetin and fiber, which support metabolic health and lower blood sugar responses.
- **Rutabaga (all forms)** — Low GI, low GL. Nutrient-rich with potassium, fiber, and vitamin C, making it a favorable substitute for higher GI root vegetables.
- **Sweet Potatoes (all forms)** — Moderate GI, moderate GL depending on cooking method. High in fiber and vitamins A and C, which help modulate blood sugar.
- **Tomatoes (all forms)** — Low GI, low GL. Rich in lycopene,

vitamin C, and potassium, tomatoes are highly beneficial for heart health and blood sugar management.

- **Winter Squash (all forms)** — Moderate GI, low GL when consumed in controlled portions. It is a great source of vitamins A and C, fiber, and antioxidants, which are all helpful for blood sugar regulation.

Beans, Peas, Lentils

- **Beans (All Cooked from Dry)**: Beans provide a variety of low glycemic load (GL) options because of their high fiber and protein content, which helps in regulating blood sugar levels.
- **Peas (All Cooked from Dry)**: Like beans, peas provide a good source of protein and fiber, contributing to blood sugar stability and supporting a low GL diet.
- **Chickpeas (Garbanzo Beans) (All Cooked from Dry)**: High in both fiber and protein, chickpeas can help manage blood sugar levels effectively.
- **Lentils (All Cooked from Dry)**: Lentils are especially beneficial in a diabetes diet as they have one of the lowest glycemic indices among legumes and are rich in fiber and protein.
- **Black Beans (All Cooked from Dry)**: Known for their deep color and rich flavor, black beans also offer antioxidant benefits alongside fiber and protein.
- **Black-Eyed Peas (All Cooked from Dry)**: These beans are particularly high in potassium and fiber, aiding in cardiovascular and glycemic health.
- **Bayo Beans (All Cooked from Dry)**: A lesser-known variety, Bayo beans are nutritious and have similar benefits to more common beans, including stabilizing blood glucose levels.
- **Cannellini Beans (All Cooked from Dry)**: These white

kidney beans are excellent for blood sugar control due to their high fiber content and protein.

- **Great Northern Beans (All Cooked from Dry)**: Another bean variety that is effective at managing blood sugar due to its low GI and high fiber.
- **Edamame (All Cooked from Dry)**: Young soybeans that are a great source of protein and fiber, making them ideal for diabetes management.
- **Kidney Beans (All Cooked from Dry)**: Rich in various nutrients including magnesium and potassium, kidney beans are effective in a low GL diet.
- **Lima Beans (All Cooked from Dry)**: Known for their buttery texture, lima beans are a good source of fiber and slow-digesting carbohydrates.
- **Mung Beans (All Cooked from Dry)**: These small green beans are packed with essential nutrients and have minimal effect on blood sugar levels.
- **Pigeon Peas (All Cooked from Dry)**: Common in tropical regions, pigeon peas are used in many traditional dishes and support glycemic control with their high fiber and protein content.
- **Pinto Beans (All Cooked from Dry)**: Popular in Mexican cuisine, pinto beans are versatile and beneficial for blood sugar regulation.
- **Split Peas (All Cooked from Dry)**: A staple in soup, split peas are highly nutritious, offering both fiber and protein to maintain stable blood glucose levels.

Starchy Vegetables

- **Breadfruit (All Fresh or Frozen)**: Rich in carbohydrates and fiber, breadfruit can be a part of a balanced diabetes diet when portion control is practiced.

- **Burdock Root (All Fresh or Frozen)**: Recognized for its earthy flavor, this food is low in calories yet high in fiber, which aids in managing blood sugar levels.
- **Cassava (All Fresh or Frozen)**: Also known as yuca, cassava is high in carbohydrates and should be consumed in moderation. It offers a gluten-free starch alternative but is low in protein and other nutrients.
- **Jicama (All Fresh or Frozen)**: Low in calories and high in fiber, jicama can be a crunchy, satisfying addition to a diabetes-friendly diet.
- **Lotus Root (All Fresh or Frozen)**: Offers a moderate amount of fiber and is rich in nutrients such as vitamin C and potassium. Its unique texture makes it versatile in cooking.
- **Plantains (All Fresh or Frozen)**: Similar to bananas but higher in starch, plantains must be cooked before eating and are best consumed in controlled portions to manage their impact on blood sugar.
- **Salsify (All Fresh or Frozen)**: Often referred to as the oyster plant due to its flavor, salsify is high in fiber and can be beneficial for blood sugar control.
- **Taro Root (Dasheen or Yautia) (All Fresh or Frozen)**: Rich in fiber and other nutrients, taro root has a lower glycemic index than many other starchy vegetables, making it suitable for a diabetes diet when used in moderation.
- **Water Chestnuts (All Fresh or Frozen)**: Though they are higher in carbohydrates, their crunchy texture and high water content make them less calorie-dense and can be included in small amounts in a diabetes-friendly diet.
- **Yam (All Fresh or Frozen)**: Yams are a good source of fiber and antioxidants, although they are higher in carbohydrates. They should be eaten in moderation within a diabetes diet.
- **Yucca (All Fresh or Frozen)**: Similar to cassava, yucca provides a high-energy carbohydrate source but lacks significant amounts of protein or fat, making it important to balance it with other nutrients.

1.6 Other Vegetables

- **Asparagus** (all fresh, frozen, cooked, or raw)
- **Avocado** (all fresh, frozen, cooked, or raw)
- **Bamboo shoots** (all fresh, frozen, cooked, or raw)
- **Beets** (all fresh, frozen, cooked, or raw)
- **Bitter melon** (all fresh, frozen, cooked, or raw)
- **Brussels sprouts** (all fresh, frozen, cooked, or raw)
- **Green cabbage** (all fresh, frozen, cooked, or raw)
- **Savoy cabbage** (all fresh, frozen, cooked, or raw)
- **Red cabbage** (all fresh, frozen, cooked, or raw)
- **Cactus pads** (all fresh, frozen, cooked, or raw)
- **Cauliflower** (all fresh, frozen, cooked, or raw)
- **Celery** (all fresh, frozen, cooked, or raw)
- **Chayote (mirliton)** (all fresh, frozen, cooked, or raw)
- **Cucumber** (all fresh, frozen, cooked, or raw)
- **Eggplant** (all fresh, frozen, cooked, or raw)
- **Green beans** (all fresh, frozen, cooked, or raw)
- **Kohlrabi** (all fresh, frozen, cooked, or raw)
- **Luffa** (all fresh, frozen, cooked, or raw)
- **Mushrooms** (all fresh, frozen, cooked, or raw)
- **Okra** (all fresh, frozen, cooked, or raw)
- **Onions** (all fresh, frozen, cooked, or raw)
- **Radish** (all fresh, frozen, cooked, or raw)
- **Rutabaga** (all fresh, frozen, cooked, or raw)
- **Seaweed** (all fresh, frozen, cooked, or raw)
- **Snow peas** (all fresh, frozen, cooked, or raw)
- **Summer squash** (all fresh, frozen, cooked, or raw)
- **Tomatillos** (all fresh, frozen, cooked, or raw)

21

THE FRUITS DIABETES-FRIENDLY FOOD LISTS

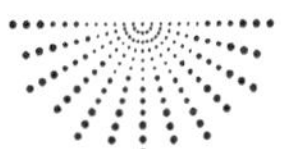

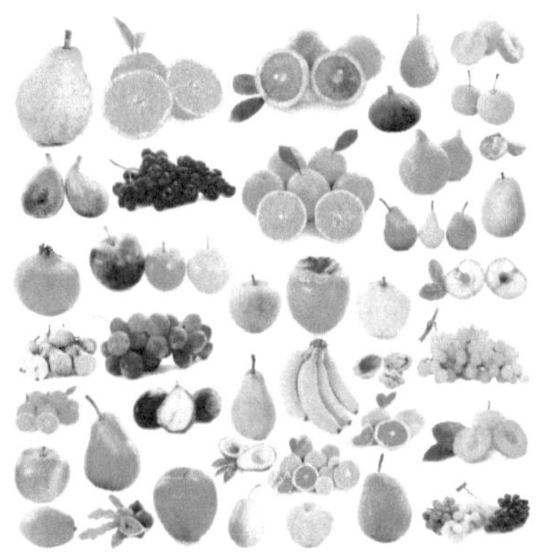

THE FRUIT FOOD GROUP AND THE LOW GL DIABETES DIET

In line with MyPlate.gov's classification, the fruit group includes all forms of fruits, such as whole fruits—whether fresh, frozen, or dried—canned fruits and 100% fruit juices. For those adhering to a low Glycemic Load (GL) diabetes diet, the focus is on whole fruits, which should constitute at least 85% of daily fruit intake in place of juices or processed fruit products. This is because whole fruits typically have lower GL values and offer a higher nutrient profile, essential for managing diabetes effectively.

NUTRIENT DENSITY AND BENEFITS OF WHOLE FRUITS

Whole fruits are nutrient-rich, providing abundant essential nutrients with relatively few calories. They're excellent sources of vitamins and minerals like vitamin C, potassium, and folate and offer phytochemicals such as phenols and antioxidants. These compounds are instrumental in reducing oxidative stress and inflammation, crucial for tackling chronic conditions like diabetes.

- **Phenolic Compounds**: These antioxidants in fruits protect cells from damage.
- **Fiber Content**: Fiber, particularly abundant in whole fruits, slows sugar absorption and lowers the glycemic response.
- **Caloric Impact**: Whole fruits have fewer calories than processed fruit products, supporting weight management—an essential aspect of diabetes care.

FRUIT JUICE AND SMOOTHIES

While 100% fruit juice is classified as fruit, it's advisable to limit its intake in the low-GL diabetes diet due to its higher GL and lack of fiber, which is vital for moderating glucose absorption. Smoothies, however, can be part of a nutritious diabetes diet if prepared with whole fruits and vegetables and other low-GL ingredients. By adding protein and healthy fats, smoothies achieve a balanced macronutrient profile that can help stabilize blood glucose.

CITRUS ADDITIONS AND FRUIT COCKTAILS

Adding citrus fruits to juices or smoothies can lower their GL due to their vitamin C and flavonoid content, which offer both metabolic benefits and antioxidant properties. The GL of a fruit cocktail, however, depends on the choice of fruits and their preparation. Fresh fruit salads and those in water instead of syrup are preferable to minimize the glycemic response.

PORTION SIZES AND INTAKE RECOMMENDATIONS

For individuals with diabetes, managing fruit intake is critical due to the natural sugars present in fruits, which can impact blood sugar levels. Adhering to recommended serving sizes is essential to ensure that each serving contains at most 15 grams of carbohydrates, aligning with diabetes management goals.

GUIDELINES FOR FRUIT INTAKE FOR DIABETES MANAGEMENT:

Carbohydrate Management: Each fruit serving is strategically sized to provide about 15 grams of carbohydrates, facilitating better blood sugar control.

Daily Recommendations: Adults are generally advised to consume at least 1.5 to 2 cups of low-GL fruit per day as part of a balanced diet.

Here's a table summarizing the serving sizes for fruits, each designed to contain no more than 15 grams of carbohydrates, alongside the general daily recommendation:

Fruit Type	Serving Size	Carbohydrate Content (Approx.)	Daily Recommended Servings
Whole Fruit (small)	1 piece (e.g., an apple, orange)	15 grams	2 servings
Berries or Melons	1 cup (raw)	15 grams	2 servings
Dried Fruit	2 tablespoons	15 grams	1 serving
100% Fruit Juice	1/2 cup	15 grams	1 serving

For fruits that are naturally larger in size or have a higher water content, such as mango, papaya, watermelon, and melon, the serving sizes should indeed be adjusted to align with the low-GL diabetes diet. Since these fruits do not share a uniform nutritional profile, tailoring the serving sizes is essential to achieve the desired carbohydrate content.

Fruit Type	Serving Size	Total Carbohydrate Content	Fiber Content	Net Carbohydrate Content	Approximate Serving for 15g of Carbohydrates
Mango	1 cup (sliced, 165g)	28 grams	3 grams	25 grams	About 1/2 cup (82.5g)
Watermelon	1 cup (diced, 152g)	11.5 grams	0.5 grams	11 grams	Slightly more than 1 cup (165g)
Papaya	1 cup (cubed, 140g)	16 grams	2.5 grams	13.5 grams	Close to 1 cup (140g)
Melon (Cantaloupe)	1 cup (cubed, 160g)	13 grams	1.4 grams	11.6 grams	Slightly more than 1 cup (170g)
Honeydew Melon	1 cup (cubed, 170g)	15 grams	1.3 grams	13.7 grams	1 cup (170g)

Mango, which is higher in carbohydrates, should be consumed in a smaller portion size than watermelon, which has fewer carbohydrates per cup and therefore allows for a larger portion. This strategy helps keep the serving size within approximately 15 grams of carbohydrates. Similarly, with careful portioning, fruits like papaya, cantaloupe, and honeydew melon can be included in the diet in amounts close to 1 cup to align with the same carbohydrate target. Adjusting serving sizes for these fruits ensures they all fit within the low GL diabetes framework, emphasizing the importance of portion control.

KEY POINTS:

Whole Fruits: Opting for whole fruits with skins provides additional fiber, which helps manage blood sugar spikes and crashes by slowing down the absorption of sugar.

Berries and Melons: These fruits are typically lower in carbohydrates per volume, allowing a more substantial portion size that contributes to satiety without significantly impacting blood sugar levels.

Dried Fruits and Juices: Due to their concentrated sugar content, these should be consumed in much smaller quantities. It's essential to check the labels for added sugars and choose unsweetened varieties wherever possible.

NATIONAL INTAKE RECOMMENDATIONS:

Underconsumption Issue: A significant portion of the American population does not meet the daily fruit intake recommendations. This shortfall can lead to a lack of essential nutrients and antioxidants that fruits provide, vital for reducing the likelihood of chronic diseases and supporting overall health.

It's essential to monitor fruit consumption closely, choosing portions and types that fit within the carbohydrate management framework. Increasing the intake of fruits not only assists in managing diabetes through controlled portions but also boosts overall health by providing necessary vitamins, minerals, and dietary fiber. Achieving the recommended daily servings of fruits can contribute to a more balanced diet and better health outcomes.

The Low-GL Diabetes Diet List

- **Apples (all fresh, frozen, dried fruits or 100% fruit juices) —**

Low GI, good fiber content, carb content: low. Apples are rich in fiber, vitamin E, C, and antioxidants, which are crucial for oxidative stress reduction and immune support. Best consumed with the skin on for maximum fiber benefit.

- **Acai (all fresh, frozen, dried fruits or 100% fruit juices)** — Generally low GI, low GL, high in antioxidants, carb content: low to moderate. Acai berries are celebrated for their profound antioxidant levels and fiber, which aid in heart health and digestion.
- **Acerola (all fresh, frozen, dried fruits or 100% fruit juices)** — Low GI, very high in vitamin C, carb content: low. Acerola cherries are an exceptional source of vitamin C, enhancing immune function and skin health.
- **Apricots (all fresh, frozen, dried fruits or 100% fruit juices)** — Low GI, especially when fresh. High in vitamins A and C, and a good source of fiber, carb content: low. Apricots support vision health and immune function.
- **Asian Pears (all fresh, frozen, dried fruits or 100% fruit juices)** — Low to moderate GI, good fiber content, carb content: low. These pears offer a juicy and refreshing taste with a mild sweet flavor, beneficial for hydration and satiety.
- **Avocados (all fresh, frozen, dried fruits or 100% fruit juices)** — Very low GI, high in healthy fats, carb content: very low. Avocados are also rich in fiber and vitamins C, E, K, and B-6, supporting cardiovascular health and weight management.
- **Blackberries (all fresh, frozen, dried fruits or 100% fruit juices)** — Very low GI, high in dietary fiber, vitamins C and K, and antioxidants, carb content: low. Blackberries contribute to heart health and cancer prevention.
- **Blueberries (all fresh, frozen, dried fruits or 100% fruit juices)** — Low to moderate GI, rich in antioxidants and fiber, carb content: low. Blueberries are known for enhancing brain health and reducing the risk of diabetes.
- **Boysenberry (all fresh, frozen, dried fruits or 100% fruit**

juices) — Low GI, high in fiber and vitamins, carb content: moderate. Known for their deep flavor, boysenberries aid in digestive health and sustain stable blood sugar levels.

- **Calamondin (all fresh, frozen, dried fruits or 100% fruit juices)** — Low GI, carb content: low. Rich in vitamin C, these are great for tropical flavored dishes and provide immune support.
- **Cantaloupe (all fresh, frozen, dried fruits or 100% fruit juices)** — Low to moderate GI, rich in vitamins A and C, hydrating, and has a high water content, carb content: moderate. Cantaloupe aids in skin health and hydration.
- **Cherimoya (all fresh, frozen, dried fruits or 100% fruit juices)** — Moderate GI, carb content: high. Rich in vitamin C and dietary fiber, cherimoya supports digestive health and immune function.
- **Cherries (all fresh, frozen, dried fruits or 100% fruit juices)** — Low GI, good source of fiber, vitamin C, and anthocyanins, carb content: moderate. Cherries are beneficial for joint health and sleep improvement.
- **Coconut (all fresh, frozen, dried fruits or 100% fruit juices)** — Low GI, high in medium-chain fatty acids, carb content: low. Coconut supports metabolism and provides a quick source of energy.
- **Cranberry (all fresh, frozen, dried fruits or 100% fruit juices)** — Low GI, carb content: low. Cranberries are high in vitamin C and are particularly beneficial for urinary tract health.
- **Currant (all fresh, frozen, dried fruits or 100% fruit juices)** — Low GI, carb content: moderate. Currants are rich in antioxidants and vitamin C, which support immune function and overall health.
- **Damson Plum (all fresh, frozen, dried fruits or 100% fruit juices)** — Low GI, carb content: moderate. Damson plums are a rich source of fiber and vitamins (A, C, and E), helpful for digestive health.

- **Durian (all fresh, frozen, dried fruits or 100% fruit juices)** — High GI, carb content: high. Known for its substantial fiber and vitamin content, durian should be consumed in moderation due to its higher carbohydrate content.
- **Grapefruit (all fresh, frozen, dried fruits or 100% fruit juices)** — Low GI, high in vitamin C and soluble fiber, carb content: low. Grapefruit can aid in cholesterol management and supports cardiovascular health.
- **Guava (all fresh, frozen, dried fruits or 100% fruit juices)** — Low GI, extremely rich in dietary fiber, vitamins A and C, carb content: moderate. Guava provides more than three times the daily recommended intake of vitamin C per fruit, enhancing immune defense and skin health.
- **Honeydew Melon (all fresh, frozen, dried fruits or 100% fruit juices)** — Low GI, provides a good source of vitamin C and is hydrating with its high water content, carb content: moderate. Honeydew is ideal for hydration and providing a quick, refreshing snack.
- **Huckleberries (all fresh, frozen, dried fruits or 100% fruit juices)** — Low GI, carb content: low. Huckleberries are high in antioxidants and fiber, promoting cardiovascular health and blood sugar regulation.
- **Jujube (all fresh, frozen, dried fruits or 100% fruit juices)** — Moderate GI, carb content: high. Jujubes are known for their high vitamin C content, supporting immune health and stress reduction.
- **Kiwifruit (all fresh, frozen, dried fruits or 100% fruit juices)** — Low to moderate GI, high in vitamins C and K, and fiber, carb content: moderate. Kiwifruit aids in digestion and boosts immune system function.
- **Lemonquat (all fresh, frozen, dried fruits or 100% fruit juices)** — Low GI, carb content: low. This hybrid fruit is rich in vitamin A, B9, C and provides a tangy addition to various dishes while supporting immune health.

- **Limes (all fresh, frozen, dried fruits or 100% fruit juices)** — Low GI, carb content: low. High in vitamin B6, B9, C and antioxidants, limes are excellent for enhancing flavor in dishes without adding sugar.
- **Lychee (all fresh, frozen, dried fruits or 100% fruit juices)** — High GI, carb content: high. Rich in vitamin C, lychee should be consumed in the recommended serving size due to its high sugar content.
- **Mangoes (all fresh, frozen, dried fruits or 100% fruit juices)** — Low GI (54), high in carbohydrates. Mangoes are abundant in vitamins A, B6, C, and fiber, which help supporting immune function and digestive health.
- **Mulberries (all fresh, frozen, dried fruits or 100% fruit juices)** — Low GI, moderate carbohydrate content. They are rich in vitamins C, B6, K, manganese and iron, beneficial for maintaining healthy blood and antioxidant levels.
- **Nectarines (all fresh, frozen, dried fruits or 100% fruit juices)** — Low GI, moderate carbohydrate content. Nectarines are a good source of vitamins A, C, E and K similar to peaches, and are great for skin health and immune support.
- **Olives (all fresh, frozen, dried fruits or 100% fruit juices)** — Low GI, low in carbohydrates but high in healthy fats, particularly oleic acid, which is good for heart health.
- **Oranges (all fresh, frozen, dried fruits or 100% fruit juices)** — Moderate GI, rich in vitamin C, potassium, and fiber, with a moderate carbohydrate content. Oranges support immune health and aid in digestive wellness.
- **Papaya (all fresh, frozen, dried fruits or 100% fruit juices)** — Moderate GI, rich in vitamins A, C, and E. High in fiber and water content, making it excellent for hydration and digestive health, with moderate carbohydrate content.
- **Peaches (all fresh, frozen, dried fruits or 100% fruit juices)** — Low GI when fresh, containing vitamins A and C along with fiber. The carbohydrate content ranges from low

to moderate, supporting overall health without spiking blood sugar levels.

- **Pears (all fresh, frozen, dried fruits or 100% fruit juices)** — Low GI, high in fiber which assists in gradual sugar absorption, with moderate carbohydrate content. Pears help maintain steady blood sugar levels.
- **Persimmon (all fresh, frozen, dried fruits or 100% fruit juices)** — Moderate to high GI, high in carbohydrates. They are rich in fiber and vitamins, promoting digestive health and providing nutritional benefits.
- **Pineapple (all fresh, frozen, dried fruits or 100% fruit juices)** — Medium GI, but rich in vitamins C and manganese, with high carbohydrate content. Pineapple is great for immune support and antioxidant protection.
- **Plums (all fresh, frozen, dried fruits or 100% fruit juices)** — Low GI, moderate carbohydrate content. When dried (prunes), they retain their fiber and nutrients, aiding in blood sugar control and digestive health.
- **Pomegranate (all fresh, frozen, dried fruits or 100% fruit juices)** — Moderate GI, high in antioxidants and vitamins, with moderate carbohydrate content. Pomegranate helps improve heart health and reduces inflammation.
- **Raspberries (all fresh, frozen, dried fruits or 100% fruit juices)** — Very low GI, low in carbohydrates, high in dietary fiber, vitamins C, and manganese. Raspberries are excellent for maintaining stable blood sugar and providing antioxidant protection.
- **Rhubarb (all fresh, frozen, dried fruits or 100% fruit juices)** — Low GI, low carbohydrate content. Known for its high vitamin K content, rhubarb supports bone health and blood clotting processes.
- **Sapote (all fresh, frozen, dried fruits or 100% fruit juices)** — Moderate GI, moderate carbohydrate content. Rich in vitamins and minerals, especially vitamin B6, C, E sapote supports immune health and provides essential nutrients.

- **Soursop (all fresh, frozen, dried fruits or 100% fruit juices)** — Moderate GI, moderate carbohydrate content. Known for its unique flavor and high vitamins and minerals content, soursop is good for immune support and cellular health.
- **Strawberries (all fresh, frozen, dried fruits or 100% fruit juices)** — Low GI, high in fiber, vitamins C, and manganese, with low carbohydrate content. Strawberries support heart health and blood sugar control.
- **Tangerines (Mandarins) (all fresh, frozen, dried fruits or 100% fruit juices)** — Low to moderate GI, low GL. Thangerines are good source of vitamins (A, C, B6, thiamin, folate) and fiber, with moderate carbohydrate content. Tangerines contribute to immune defense and digestive health.
- **Watermelon (all fresh, frozen, dried fruits or 100% fruit juices)** — Despite its high GI, watermelon has a low glycemic load due to its high water content, rich in vitamins (A, B6, C, folate) with moderate carbohydrate content. Watermelon is excellent for hydration and providing essential nutrients.

22
THE GRAINS DIABETES-FRIENDLY FOOD LISTS

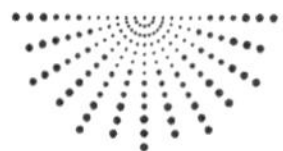

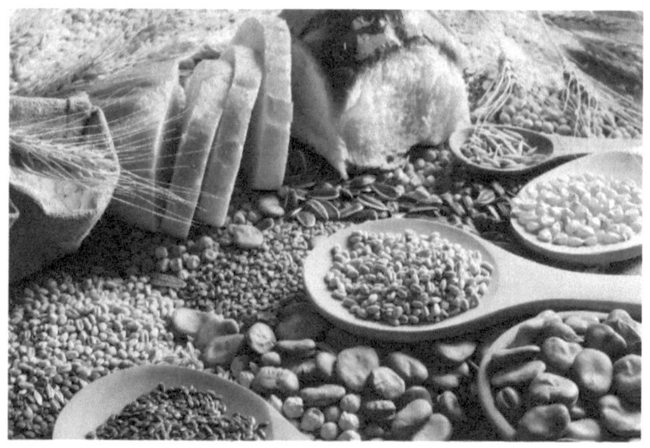

Aligned with the classification system from MyPlate.gov, the grains group encompasses all forms of grains, including whole grains (such as whole wheat, brown rice, and quinoa) and refined grains (like white rice and white flour). For individuals adhering to the low GL diabetes diet, the emphasis is on whole grains, which should constitute the majority of daily grain intake. This is because whole grains generally have lower GL values and provide a richer nutrient profile.

NUTRIENT DENSITY AND BENEFITS OF WHOLE GRAINS

Whole grains are densely packed with nutrients, providing abundant vital nutrients while maintaining a low-calorie content. They are excellent sources of:

- **Complex Carbohydrates and Dietary Fibers:** Slowly digested, these help sustain stable blood sugar levels and enhance satiety.
- **B Vitamins:** These nutrients are crucial for a range of metabolic functions, such as generating energy and forming red blood cells.
- **Minerals:** Including iron for blood health, magnesium for muscle and nerve function, and selenium for immune support.

Experts advise incorporating a minimum of three servings of whole grains into your daily diet, equating to about 15-20 grams of total carbohydrates or 15 grams of net carbohydrates, aligning with low-GL diabetes diet recommendations.

CALCULATED PORTION SIZES FOR VARIOUS WHOLE GRAINS

To meet these dietary guidelines, the following portion sizes are recommended:

- **Porridge Oats**: 23 to 30 grams
- **Muesli**: 25 to 30 grams
- **Toasted Whole Grain Oat Cereal**: 20 to 27 grams
- **Multi-grain Bread**: 1 slice (31 to 42 grams per slice)
- **Brown Rice**: 65 to 87 grams (cooked)
- **Wholewheat Pasta**: 60 to 80 grams (cooked)
- **Wholewheat Bread**: 1 slice (33 to 44 grams per slice)
- **Rye Bread**: 1 slice (31 to 42 grams per slice)

- **Barley Bread**: 1 slice (33 to 44 grams per slice, similar to wholewheat bread)
- **Bran Cereal**: 23 to 31 grams
- **Cooked Cereal (e.g., wheat, oats)**: 75 to 100 grams (cooked)
- **Barley**: 54 to 71 grams (cooked)
- **Buckwheat**: 75 to 100 grams (cooked)
- **Quinoa**: 71 to 95 grams (cooked)
- **Amaranth**: 65 to 87 grams (cooked)
- **Teff**: 75 to 100 grams (cooked)
- **Bulgur**: 83 to 111 grams (cooked)
- **Sorghum**: 60 to 80 grams (cooked)
- **Millet**: 65 to 87 grams (cooked)
- **Wild Rice**: 71 to 95 grams (cooked)
- **Triticale**: 75 to 100 grams (cooked)

WHOLE GRAINS AND DIABETES MANAGEMENT:

The evidence strongly supports the inclusion of whole grains in the low-GL Diabetes Diet as part of effective diabetes management. Regular consumption of whole grains, particularly types like oats, known for their beneficial effects on glycemic markers, can play a crucial role in controlling diabetes and improving overall health.

Research indicates that whole grains can enhance insulin sensitivity and decrease blood sugar following meals. Studies consistently show that diets rich in whole grains can significantly improve fasting blood glucose, fasting insulin, glycated hemoglobin (HbA1c), and insulin resistance compared to diets high in refined grains or low in whole grains.

Here's a synthesis of the findings from several research studies on the topic:

- **Whole Grains and Diabetes Management**: The consumption of whole grains is linked to a reduced likelihood of developing type 2 diabetes. This relationship is attributed to whole grains' ability to improve insulin sensitivity and reduce postprandial blood glucose levels. A comprehensive review and meta-analysis found that higher intake of whole grains is linked to significant reductions in fasting glucose, fasting insulin, glycated hemoglobin (HbA1c), and insulin resistance measures when compared with refined grains or non-whole grain consumption.

- **Specific Whole Grains**: Different whole grains, such as oats, brown rice, and wheat, have been studied for their effects on glycemic control. Oats, in particular, have been highlighted for their significantly beneficial impact on glycemic markers compared to other grains. This suggests that the type of whole grain consumed may also affect diabetes management.
- **Mechanisms**: The positive effects of whole grains on diabetes management are thought to be due to their high fiber content, which can slow glucose absorption into the bloodstream, thus lowering postprandial blood glucose and insulin levels. Additionally, whole grains contain bioactive compounds that may improve insulin sensitivity.
- **Quantity and Frequency**: The beneficial effects of whole grains on glycemic control appear to be dose-dependent, with greater intakes associated with more significant improvements. Regular consumption of whole grains is recommended for sustained benefits in diabetes management.

THE "FREE GRAIN DIET" FOR DIABETES

The "Free Grain Diet" for diabetes, or any diet suggesting the complete avoidance of grains, has its share of criticisms and potential pitfalls. While some proponents argue that eliminating grains can aid control blood sugar levels, enhance insulin sensitivity, and reduce inflammation, there are several considerations and criticisms to bear in mind:

Nutritional Deficiencies: Whole grains are a significant source of essential nutrients, including dietary fiber, B vitamins, iron, magnesium, phosphorus, manganese, and selenium. Removing them from the diet might lead to nutrient deficiencies, requiring careful planning or supplementation to avoid adverse health consequences.

Fiber Intake: Whole grains provide ample dietary fiber, essential for digestive well-being, aiding in blood sugar regulation, and linked to a reduced risk of cardiovascular issues. A diet devoid of whole grains may lead to insufficient fiber intake, potentially causing digestive issues such as constipation and negatively affecting heart health.

Impact on Gut Health: Dietary grain fibers act as prebiotics, feeding beneficial gut bacteria. Reducing these fibers can adversely affect the diversity and overall health of the gut microbiome, which is linked to various health outcomes, including immune function and mental health.

Unsustainable and Restrictive: Diets that strictly limit whole categories of foods can be challenging to maintain long-term and may lead to an unhealthy relationship with food. The restriction can make it hard for individuals to stick to the diet, potentially leading to cycles of restriction and binge eating.

Overemphasis on Grain Elimination: Focusing solely on eliminating grains might overlook the importance of a balanced diet that includes a variety of foods. Managing diabetes effectively involves considering the overall quality of the diet, including the intake of sugars, fats, and processed foods, rather than targeting a single food group.

Lack of Long-term Evidence: There is limited long-term research on the effects of entirely grain-free diets on diabetes management. While low-carbohydrate diets are beneficial in managing type 2 diabetes in the short term, the long-term health impacts of altogether avoiding grains are unclear.

Generalization Issues: People with diabetes have individual responses to different foods, including grains. What might work for one person regarding blood sugar management might not work for another.

THE LOW-GL DIABETES DIET LIST

Here is a detailed list of whole grains and pseudo-grains with an emphasis on ensuring each recommended serving size contains about 15 grams of carbohydrates, typically aligning with a low GL:

Whole Grains

- **Barley** — Low GL for the recommended serving size, which provides substantial fiber aiding in slow glucose absorption.
- **Brown Rice** — Low to moderate GL, when portioned correctly, supports steady energy with its complex carbohydrates.
- **Bulgur** — Low GL at proper serving sizes, known for quick preparation and maintaining blood sugar levels.
- **Millet** — Naturally gluten-free with a low GL, offers versatile uses in a diabetic diet.
- **Oats (Avena sativa L.)** — Low GL, especially when consumed as steel-cut or old-fashioned oats, beneficial for heart and glycemic health.
- **Dark Rye** — Low GL when eaten in appropriate portions, denser and more filling which helps in managing hunger and blood sugar.
- **Whole Wheat Bread** — Moderate GL, selecting high-fiber varieties ensures better glycemic control.
- **Whole Wheat Chapati** — Moderate GL, provides sustained energy release when eaten in controlled amounts.
- **Whole Grain Cereals** — The GL varies; choosing less processed options with no added sugars keeps the GL low.
- **Wild Rice** — Low GL, offers a nutritious alternative to traditional white rice with more protein and fiber.

- **Sorghum** — Low GL, this versatile, gluten-free grain can be popped like popcorn or used as a rice substitute.
- **Triticale** — Low to moderate GL, combines the qualities of wheat and rye for a nutrient-rich grain choice.
- **Pseudo-grains**
- **Buckwheat** — Low GL, provides a hearty, nutritious option for breakfast porridge or as a rice substitute.
- **Quinoa** — Low GL for the recommended serving, complete protein that's ideal for vegetarian diets.
- **Amaranth** — Low GL, this protein-rich pseudo-grain is excellent for porridge or added to soups and stews.
- **Spelt** — Moderate GL, spelt offers a nutty flavor and can replace wheat in most recipes.
- **Kamut** — Low GL, known for its rich, buttery flavor and higher protein content compared to regular wheat.
- **Teff** — Low GL, highly nutritious, ideal for making porridge or gluten-free baked goods.

These grains and pseudo-grains should be incorporated into meals in measured amounts to maintain a low GL, supporting effective diabetes management through controlled blood sugar levels. Each grain can contribute to a balanced diet, enhancing overall health while providing essential nutrients and energy.

23
THE DAIRY AND PLANT-BASED ALTERNATIVES DIABETES-FRIENDLY FOOD LISTS

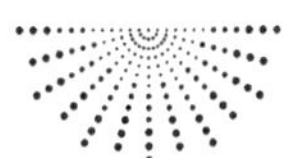

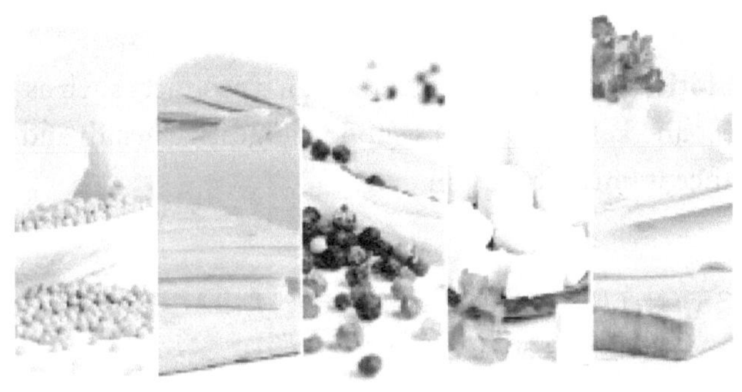

THE DAIRY AND PLANT-BASED ALTERNATIVES GROUP IN THE LOW GL DIABETES DIET

Aligned with MyPlate.gov's classification, the dairy group encompasses all forms of dairy products, including milk, cheese, yogurt, and butter, as well as plant-based alternatives like almond milk, soy milk, and coconut yogurt. For individuals following the low-GL diabetes diet, the emphasis is on choosing options with minimal added sugars and high in calcium and other essential nutrients.

NUTRIENT DENSITY AND BENEFITS OF DAIRY AND PLANT-BASED ALTERNATIVES

Dairy products and their plant-based alternatives can be nutrient-rich, providing essential nutrients with varying calorie contents. They serve as excellent sources of calcium, vitamin D, and protein, providing added health advantages.

- **Calcium and Vitamin D**: Crucial for bone health, these nutrients help prevent osteoporosis and support muscle function.
- **Protein**: Essential for adequate muscle repair and growth, protein also helps regulate blood sugar by slowing the digestion of carbohydrates.
- **Probiotics**: Present in fermented dairy products such as yogurt and kefir, probiotics support digestive health and can enhance immune function.

CHOICES IN THE DAIRY AND PLANT-BASED ALTERNATIVES GROUP

1. **Milk and Milk Alternatives**: Unsweetened versions of soy, almond, and oat milk provide low-GL options that are high in vitamins and minerals.
2. **Cheese**: Opt for natural cheeses. While these contain minimal carbohydrates, they should be used sparingly due to their elevated saturated fat content.
3. **Yogurt**: Unsweetened, plain yogurt, especially Greek yogurt,

is recommended due to its lower carbohydrate content and higher protein level.

4. **Butter and Cream**: While these contain minimal carbohydrates, they should be used sparingly due to their high saturated fat content.

Dairy and Smoothies

Incorporating dairy or plant-based milk and yogurt into smoothies can add essential nutrients and help achieve a balanced macronutrient profile that can stabilize blood glucose levels. Adding sources of healthy fats, like avocado or nuts, can further improve the nutritional profile of these smoothies.

PORTION SIZES AND INTAKE RECOMMENDATIONS

For individuals with diabetes, managing the intake of dairy and dairy alternatives is crucial because even small amounts of added sugars can impact blood sugar levels. Serving sizes should be controlled to ensure minimal impact on blood glucose:

- **Carbohydrate Management**: Each serving should ideally contain less than 12 grams of carbohydrates, particularly for milk and yogurt.
- **Daily Recommendations**: Adults are generally advised to include 3 servings of dairy or plant-based alternatives each day as part of a balanced diet.

Here's a table summarizing the serving sizes for dairy and plant-based alternatives, each designed to align with low GL recommendations and diabetes management goals:

Product Type	Recommended Serving Size	Carbohydrate Content
Unsweetened Soy Milk	1 cup	3-4 grams
Unsweetened Almond Milk	1 cup	1-2 grams
Unsweetened Oat Milk	1 cup	15-19 grams
Plain Greek Yogurt	1/2 cup	5-7 grams
Natural Cheese	1 ounce	0-1 grams
Tofu	1/2 cup (cubed)	1-2 grams
Soy Yogurt (unsweetened)	1/2 cup	4-6 grams
Cottage Cheese	1/2 cup	4-5 grams

RECOMMENDATIONS FOR DAIRY AND PLANT-BASED ALTERNATIVES IN DIABETES MANAGEMENT:

- **Select Minimally Processed Options**: Opt for dairy and plant-based alternatives that are unsweetened and free from unnecessary additives. This ensures lower carbohydrate content and aligns with a low GL diet.
- **Diversify Your Choices**: Incorporate a variety of non-dairy milk, such as unsweetened soy, almond, and oat milk, to benefit from their unique nutritional profiles. Soy milk, for example, offers high protein, which is beneficial for blood sugar control.
- **Focus on Probiotic-Rich Foods**: Choose plain, unsweetened yogurt and soy yogurt containing probiotics to support gut health. These are particularly useful for diabetes management due to their impact on digestion and overall gut flora balance.
- **Adhere to Recommended Portions**: Carefully measure

servings to control carbohydrate intake, which is crucial for maintaining stable blood glucose levels. This is especially important for products like oat milk, which tend to have higher carbohydrate content.

- **Incorporate Healthy Proteins**: Tofu and cottage cheese are protein-rich foods that are low in carbohydrates. They can be excellent in various dishes and contribute to satiety and muscle maintenance without spiking blood sugar.
- **Use in Balanced Meals**: Thoughtfully integrate these dairy and plant-based alternatives into your meals. For instance, blend soy milk into smoothies, add tofu to stir-fries, or enjoy a bowl of Greek yogurt with nuts and seeds for a nutritious snack.

This approach helps ensure that each choice supports blood sugar control and overall health.

THE LOW-GL DIABETES DIET FOOD LIST

Here's a detailed breakdown of dairy and plant-based alternatives suitable for the low-GL diabetes diet:

Dairy and Plant-Based Milk Alternatives

- **Cow's Milk** — Available in fluid, evaporated, or dry forms, including lactose-free and reduced options. Cow's milk provides significant amounts of calcium, vitamin D, and protein but can vary in carbohydrate content depending on the type (whole, skim, etc.).
- **Goat's Milk** — Similar to cow's milk in nutrient profile, goat's milk provides a good alternative for those looking for different flavor profiles or digestibility. It is also available in lactose-free forms.

- **Buttermilk**—Traditionally left over after churning butter, it is now commercially produced as cultured buttermilk. It is lower in fat and calories but high in potassium and calcium and available in lactose-reduced forms.
- **Soy Milk** — A plant-based milk alternative without added sugars or additives, rich in protein and fortified with calcium and vitamins typically found in cow's milk. It has a low GI and is a good option for those avoiding dairy.
- **Almond Milk**—Made from ground almonds and water, this milk alternative is low in calories and carbohydrates, making it suitable for a low-GL diet when unsweetened.
- **Coconut Milk**—Extracted from the flesh of coconuts, this milk is rich in medium-chain triglycerides (MCTs) and usually low in carbohydrates, making it suitable for a low GL diet when unsweetened.
- **Oat Milk** — Derived from whole oat grains, it's higher in carbohydrates than some other plant-based milk but offers a good amount of fiber and is often enriched with vitamins and minerals.
- **Cashew Milk** — Similar to almond milk, cashew milk is low in carbohydrates and calories, provided it's unsweetened, making it a viable option for those monitoring their blood sugar levels.
- **Rice Milk** — Generally the highest in carbohydrates among plant milks, unsweetened rice milk can still be part of a diabetes diet if portion sizes are controlled.

Dairy and Fermented Products

- **Yogurt** — Including Greek, Bulgarian, and plain varieties, without added sugars. Rich in protein and probiotics, these yogurts support digestive health and can aid manage blood sugar levels.
- **Kefir**—A fermented milk drink similar to thin yogurt, kefir is

high in probiotics and low in lactose. It is excellent for gut health and potentially beneficial for blood sugar control.

- **Frozen Yogurt** — Often enjoyed as a dessert, choose versions without added sugars and watch portions to ensure they fit within the low GL eating pattern (15 grams of carbs at most).

Cheese Varieties

- **Cheeses**—Including natural, low-fat, and non-dairy options such as soy cheese, cheeses are generally low in carbohydrates, making them a good choice for a low-GL diet.
- **Cottage Cheese** — Low-fat versions are high in protein and low in fat, making them suitable for those managing diabetes.
- **Cream Cheese** — Low-fat and lactose-reduced varieties offer a way to enjoy this spread without significantly impacting blood sugar levels.
- **Ricotta Cheese** — Typically used in sweet and savory dishes, ricotta can be part of a diabetes-friendly diet when choosing low-fat and lactose-reduced options.

Plant-Based Proteins

- **Soy Cheese** — A non-dairy alternative low in carbohydrates and can be used similarly to dairy cheese.
- **Tempeh** — Made from fermented soybeans, tempeh is high in protein and fiber, which are beneficial for blood sugar management.
- **Tofu**—Also derived from soy, tofu is characterized by its low carbs content and high protein content, making it a favorable option for individuals following a low-glycemic load diet.

This detailed list offers a variety of dairy—and plant-based alternatives, providing options to enjoy while ensuring they maintain balanced blood sugar levels.

24

PROTEIN DIABETESDIABETES-FRIENDLY FOOD LISTS

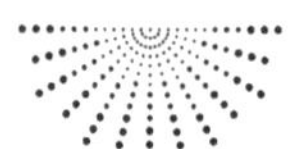

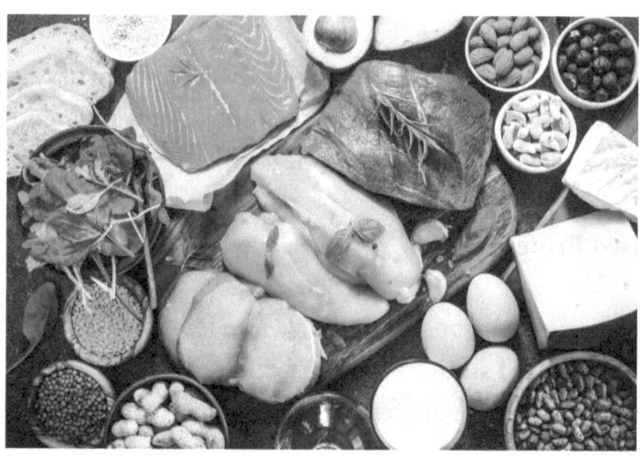

THE PROTEIN FOODS GROUP IN THE LOW GL DIABETES DIET

Aligned with MyPlate.gov's classification, the protein foods group includes a wide array of animal and plant-based sources such as meats, poultry, fish, eggs, nuts, seeds, and legumes. For individuals following a low Glycemic Load (GL) diabetes diet, the focus is on selecting lean, minimally processed options that provide essential nutrients without unnecessary additives or high levels of saturated fats.

Incorporating protein foods into meals enhances flavor and satiety and helps maintain stable blood glucose levels. Combining protein with carbohydrates in meals can help delay the absorption process of sugar into the bloodstream, preventing spikes.

NUTRIENT DENSITY AND BENEFITS OF PROTEIN FOODS

Protein foods are crucial for a balanced diet, offering more than just protein but also a variety of vital vitamins, minerals, and other beneficial compounds:

- **High-Quality Protein**: Essential for muscle repair, growth, and overall health. Protein also helps regulate blood sugar levels by promoting satiety and slowing the digestion of carbohydrates.
- **Omega-3** : Present in fatty fish such as salmon, mackerel, and sardines, omega-3s help reduce inflammation and are linked to heart health.
- **Iron and Zinc**: Meat, especially red meat, is a significant source of iron and zinc, which are vital for immune function and energy metabolism.
- **Fiber and Phytonutrients**: Plant-based proteins such as beans, lentils, and chickpeas offer fiber, which helps manage blood sugar levels, and phytonutrients that play a role in reducing chronic disease risk.

CHOICES IN THE PROTEIN FOODS GROUP

1. **Lean Meats**: Including chicken, turkey, and lean cuts of beef and pork. Opt for grilled, baked, or steamed versions without added fats or sugars.

2. **Fish and Seafood**: Emphasize fatty fish for added omega-3 fatty acids and choose fresh or frozen options prepared with minimal added fats.
3. **Eggs**: A versatile protein source that can be included in various dishes, from omelets to salads.
4. **Legumes**: Beans, chickpeas and lentils are excellent fiber-rich protein sources and are particularly beneficial in a diabetes diet.
5. **Nuts and Seeds**: Include a variety of nuts and seeds, such as cashews, walnuts, peanuts, pistachios, almonds, flaxseeds, and chia seeds, for their protein, healthy fats, and fiber.
6. **Plant-Based Proteins**: Tofu, tempeh, and edamame provide high-quality protein and other nutrients beneficial for those managing diabetes.

PORTION SIZES AND INTAKE RECOMMENDATIONS

For individuals with diabetes, managing protein intake is crucial, especially considering saturated fat content. Optimal serving sizes ensure a balanced nutrient intake without overloading on calories:

- **Protein Management**: Aim for approximately 15-25 grams of protein per meal, depending on individual dietary needs and total daily calorie intake.
- **Daily Recommendations**: Adults are generally advised to include 2-3 servings of lean protein sources each day as part of a balanced diet. However, they must meet the target dietary protein intake in all cases, as detailed in the chapter "Protein — The Building Blocks of Life."

The protein foods group consists of a variety of foods that are good protein sources. These foods include:

1. **Meat:** Beef, pork, lamb, veal, and game meats such as venison.
2. **Poultry:** Chicken, turkey, duck, and other fowl.

3. **Seafood:** Fish, shellfish, and other seafood such as shrimp, crab, and lobster.
4. **Eggs:** Chicken eggs, quail eggs, and other types of eggs.
5. **Nuts and seeds:** Almonds, peanuts, walnuts, pumpkin seeds, and sunflower seeds.

Here's a table summarizing the serving sizes for protein foods with nutritional informations:

Protein Source	Serving Size	Key Nutrients	Specific Notes
Poultry (Chicken, Turkey)	3-4 ounces	Protein, B vitamins	Ideal for general health and muscle maintenance
Fish (Salmon, Tuna, Mackerel)	3-4 ounces	Protein, omega-3 fatty acids	Supports heart health and reduces inflammation
Seafood (Shrimp, Crabs)	3-4 ounces	Protein, essential minerals	Low in fat and calories
Lean Beef	3-4 ounces	Protein, iron, zinc	Choose lean cuts to reduce intake of saturated fats
Legumes (Beans, Lentils)	1/2 cup cooked	Protein, fiber, iron	Great plant-based protein source, helps in blood sugar control
Nuts and Seeds (Almonds, Walnuts, Flaxseeds)	1/4 cup	Protein, healthy fats, fiber	Enhances satiety, good for heart health
Tofu	1/2 cup	Protein, calcium	Plant-based, suitable for those managing CKD
Eggs	1-2 eggs	Protein, vitamins D and B12	Versatile and nutrient-dense
Dairy (Cheese, Yogurt)	1 ounce (cheese), 1/2 cup (yogurt)	Protein, calcium, probiotics	Choose low-fat and unsweetened varieties for diabetes management
Plant-Based Alternatives (Tempeh, Seitan)	3-4 ounces	Protein	Suitable for vegans and those with dietary restrictions

THE LOW GL DIABETES DIET FOOD LIST

Meats, Poultry, Eggs, and Seafood Group: This group is a vital part of the diet, providing high-quality protein and essential nutrients that are crucial for health, especially in managing diabetes. Here's how each type can be integrated into a low Glycemic Load (GL) diabetes diet:

- **Beef, Lamb, Pork, Goat**: Choose lean cuts (e.g., sirloin, tenderloin) and prefer grass-fed options when possible. These meats should be consumed in moderation and cooked adequately to preserve nutrients and ensure safety. Ground versions should be at least 90% lean.
- **Game Meat (Bison, Venison, Elk, Moose)**: Naturally leaner, these meats are abundant sources of protein and iron. They should be cooked thoroughly to optimize digestibility and safety.

- **Chicken and Turkey**: Skinless options are preferred to minimize fat intake. Both can be enjoyed cooked adequately in various forms, such as roasted, grilled, or boiled. Ground chicken or turkey should be considered if it's at least 93% lean.
- **Duck and Goose**: Higher in fat, these should be consumed less frequently and with the skin removed to reduce fat content.
- **Game Birds (Ostrich, Pheasant, Quail)**: These are excellent sources of lean protein and should be cooked thoroughly to ensure safety.

- **Chicken, Duck, Turkey, and Other Birds' Eggs**: Eggs are versatile and can be consumed cooked in styles such as boiled, scrambled, or poached. They provide high-quality protein, important vitamins and minerals.

Seafood

- **Fatty Fish (Salmon, Mackerel, Sardines, Herring, Trout)**: Rich in omega-3 fatty acids, these should be included regularly in the diet. They can be consumed cooked adequately through methods like grilling or baking.
- **White Fish (Cod, Tilapia, Flounder, Sole, Pollock)**: Low in fat and high in protein, ideal for frequent consumption cooked adequately to maintain nutrient integrity.
- **Shellfish (Shrimp, Lobster, Crab, Clams, Oysters, Scallops)**: High in protein and minerals but should be consumed in moderation due to cholesterol content. Ensure they are cooked thoroughly to avoid foodborne illnesses.
- **Other Seafood (Squid, Octopus)**: These can be included and should be cooked adequately to ensure they are tender and safe to eat.

Nuts, Seeds, and Soy Products in the Low GL Diabetes Diet

This group is essential for providing healthy fats, proteins, fiber, and various micronutrients that can enhance overall health and help manage diabetes more effectively.

Nuts and Nut Butter

Nuts are a heart-healthy food group rich in unsaturated fats, proteins, vitamins, and minerals. They can be incorporated into the low GL diabetes diet in moderation due to their high caloric content:

- **Almonds**: High in vitamin E and magnesium, helpful for blood sugar control.
- **Pecans**: Rich in antioxidants and beneficial fats.
- **Brazil Nuts**: Best known for their selenium content, which supports thyroid function.
- **Pistachios**: Good for heart health, with a balance of protein and fiber.
- **Hazelnuts**: High in vitamin E and healthy fats.
- **Macadamias**: High in monounsaturated fats.

- **Pine Nuts**: Good source of iron and magnesium.
- **Walnuts**: Rich in alpha-linolenic acid, an omega-3 fatty acid.
- **Cashew Nuts**: Lower fat content than other nuts, rich in copper and magnesium.

Nut butter should be chosen carefully, ensuring it is natural and without added sugars or excessive salts.

Seeds and Seed Butter

Seeds offer similar nutritional benefits as nuts but are generally higher in fiber and contain unique beneficial compounds:

- **Pumpkin Seeds**: A good magnesium, zinc, and fatty acids source.
- **Psyllium Seeds**: These are mainly used for their fiber content, which can help digestion and aid stabilize blood sugar levels.
- **Chia Seeds**: Exceptionally high in omega-3 and fiber.
- **Flax Seeds**: High in omega-3 and lignans, which have antioxidant properties.
- **Sunflower Seeds**: Rich in vitamin B6, E, thiamine and selenium.
- **Sesame Seeds**: Good source of calcium and magnesium.
- **Poppy Seeds**: Contain calcium, iron, and zinc.

Like nut butter, seed butter (e.g., sunflower butter or tahini, made from sesame seeds) should be chosen without added sugars or salts and can be used in various culinary applications, from dressings to spreads.

Soy Products

Soy products are excellent plant-based protein sources that can be beneficial in a diabetes diet:

- **Tofu**: Versatile and can be used in savory and sweet dishes; high in protein and calcium when fortified.

- **Tempeh**: Fermented, making it richer in protein and nutrients than tofu and easier to digest.
- **Edamame**: Young soybeans are often eaten as a snack; high in protein and fiber.
- **Soy Milk**: An alternative option to dairy milk; choose unsweetened varieties to keep sugar intake low.

Integration into the Diet

Nuts, seeds, and soy products can be incorporated into the diet in various ways:

- **As a Snack**: Raw or roasted nuts and seeds are great for snacking.
- **In Meals**: Add nuts or seeds to salads, yogurt, or oatmeal for extra texture and nutrients.
- **Soy Products**: Use tofu in stir-fries, soups, and stews, or blend silken tofu into smoothies for added protein.

THE DIABETES-FRIENDLY CARBS, PROTEINS, FATS AND FIBER COUNTER

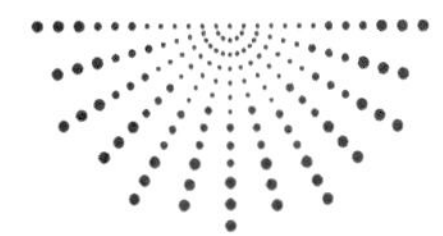

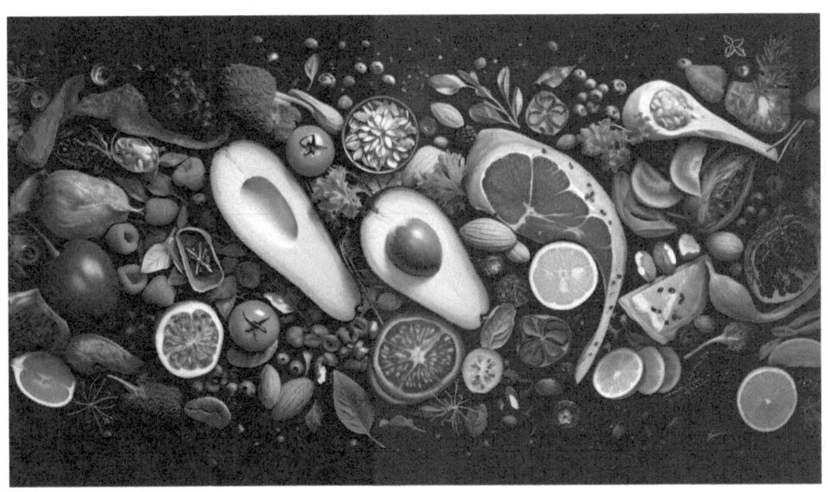

1

INTRODUCTION TO THE DIABETES-FRIENDLY CARBS, PROTEINS, FATS AND FIBER COUNTER

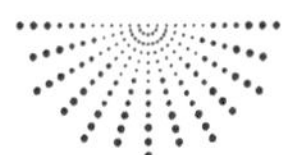

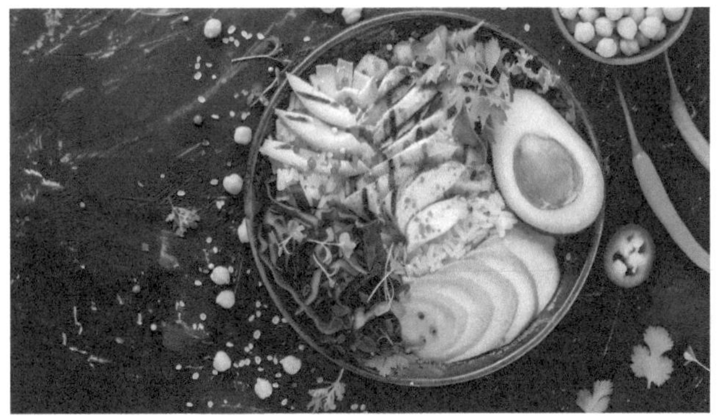

INTRODUCTION TO "THE DIABETES-FRIENDLY CARBS, PROTEINS, FATS, AND FIBER COUNTER"

This volume serves as the second tier in the Low-Glycemic Load Diabetes Diet, focusing on carefully selecting carbohydrates, proteins, fats, and fibers to support individuals managing diabetes. Each food item included has undergone a thorough evaluation to ensure compatibility with the principles of a low-GL diet, aiming to positively influence diabetes management.

The selection in this counter is designed to minimize blood sugar fluctuations. Foods are chosen for their low impact on blood glucose levels, and portions are calibrated to typically not exceed 15 grams of net carbs. Additionally, the focus on nutrient density ensures that each serving provides a maximum health benefit without excess calories. This approach aligns with the CDC guidelines, emphasizing nutrient density and controlled portion sizes in managing health.

In categories like Dairy and Plant-based Alternatives, sodium content is also provided for each serving to aid in comprehensive dietary decision-making, helping manage both carbohydrate intake and sodium levels effectively.

VOLUME STRUCTURE

The counter is systematically organized into specific categories, each outlined to facilitate easy access to essential diabetes-friendly food choices:

1. Breads & Baked Foods
2. Beans and Pulses
3. Beef, Veal, Lamb, Pork, Poultry
4. Dairy and Plant-based Alternatives
5. Fruits & Fruit Products.
6. Grains & Cereals
7. Nuts & Seeds
8. Seafood & Shellfish
9. Vegetables & Vegetable Products

This counter is a strategic tool to guide daily food choices within a structured dietary framework. It aims to equip you with detailed knowledge of the nutritional content of foods, enabling precise management of diabetes through informed dietary strategies. The categorization and detailed listings aid in simplifying dietary decision-making, helping individuals manage their diabetes confidently and effectively. This counter also reflects a commitment to adhering to established health guidelines, ensuring that each food choice supports the overall health objectives of individuals with diabetes.

USING THE COUNTER: STEP-BY-STEP GUIDE

To maximize the benefits of the Diabetes-Friendly Carbs, Proteins, Fats, and Fiber Counter, follow this step-by-step guide to make informed and healthy dietary choices:

1. **Begin with Food Group Selection:** Start by selecting a food group from the organized categories in this counter. The categories include Breads & Baked Foods, Beans and Pulses, Meats, Dairy and Alternatives, Fruits and Fruit Products, Grains and Cereals, Nuts and Seeds, Seafood and Shellfish, and Vegetables and Vegetable Products. This allows for targeted and easy navigation based on your dietary needs or preferences.
2. **Understand Serving Sizes:** For each food item, refer to the calibrated serving sizes provided. These sizes are usually designed to ensure that net carbohydrates do not exceed 15 grams per serving. This calibration is crucial for maintaining blood sugar levels within a safe range.
3. **Check Nutrient Density:** Evaluate the nutrient density of each food option. Nutrient-dense foods provide more beneficial nutrients relative to their calorie content, supporting overall health without unnecessary caloric intake.
4. **Adjust According to Dietary Guidelines:** Adjust based on specific dietary needs or goals. This may include considering sodium content for those managing blood pressure or fat content for those focusing on cardiovascular health. Use the detailed information for each food item to tailor your diet effectively.
5. **Incorporate Variety:** Ensure a balanced diet by including a variety of foods from different categories. This variety helps

cover all nutritional bases, from antioxidants in fruits and vegetables to essential fatty acids in nuts and seeds.

6. **Regular Review and Adjustment:** Review your choices regularly and make adjustments as needed based on your health outcomes or changes in dietary guidelines. This dynamic approach allows personalized diet management that evolves with your health needs.

By following these steps, you can effectively use the "Diabetes-Friendly Carbs, Proteins, Fats, and Fiber Counter" to make educated food selections that support your management of diabetes. This structured approach simplifies the process of choosing what to eat and ensures that your diet contributes positively to enhance substantially your diabetes management and overall health

2

BREADS & BAKED FOODS

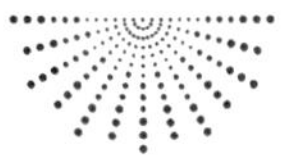

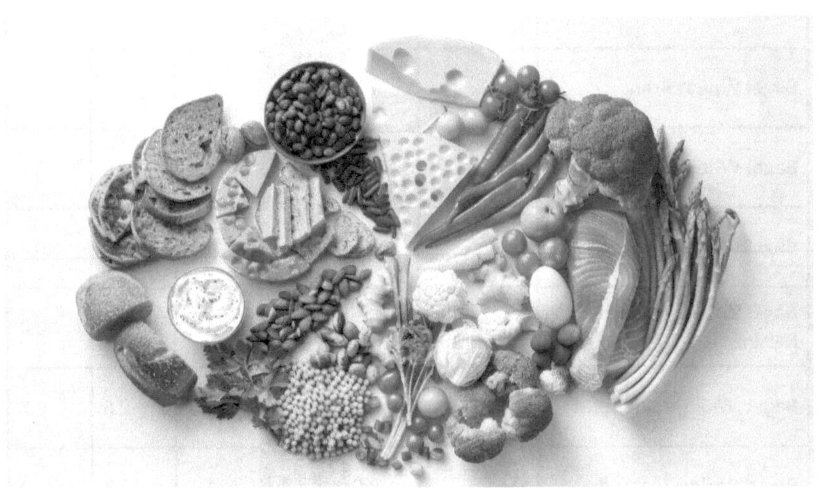

FOOD	SERVING SIZE	CALORIES	TOTAL CARB (g)	FIBER (g)	PROTEIN (g)	FAT (g)
Bagel Multigrain	1 mini, 28g	70	13.7	1.1	2.9	0.4
Bagel Multigrain with Raisins	1 mini, 28g	71	14.5	1.1	2.7	0.4
Bagel Oat Bran	1 mini, 28g	71	14.9	1	3	0.3
Bagel Oat Bran	1 mini, 28g	70	13.7	1.1	2.9	0.4
Bagel Pumpernickel	1 mini, 28g	70	13.7	1.1	2.9	0.4
Bagel Wheat	1 mini, 28g	70	13.7	1.1	2.9	0.4
Bagel Wheat Bran	1 mini, 28g	70	13.7	1.1	2.9	0.4
Bagel Whole Grain White	1 mini, 28g	70	13.7	1.1	2.9	0.4
Bagel Whole Wheat	1 mini, 28g	70	13.7	1.1	2.9	0.4
Bagel Whole Wheat with Raisins	1 mini, 28g	71	14.5	1.1	2.7	0.4
Bagels Multigrain	1 mini, 28g	67	13.3	1.7	2.8	0.3
Bread Barley Toasted	1 slice, 28g	84	14.6	1.2	3.3	1.4
Bread Black Toasted	1 slice, 28g	77	14.6	2	2.7	1

FOOD	SERVING SIZE	CALORIES	TOTAL CARB (g)	FIBER (g)	PROTEIN (g)	FAT (g)
Bread Chapati Whole Wheat	1 slice, 28g	83	13	1.4	3.2	2.1
Bread Cracked-Wheat	1 slice, 28g	73	13.9	1.5	2.4	1.1
Bread Egg Challah Toasted	1 slice, 28g	88	14.7	0.7	2.9	1.8
Bread Egg Toasted	1 slice, 28g	88	14.7	0.7	2.9	1.8
Bread Focaccia Plain	1 piece, 28g	70	10	0.5	2.5	2.2
Bread French or Vienna Whole Wheat	1 slice, 28g	67	13.7	1.2	2.3	0.3
Bread Gluten Free Toasted	1 slice, 28g	76	14.1	1.3	1.3	1.6
Bread High Protein Toasted	1 slice, 28g	75	13.5	0.9	3.7	0.7
Bread Injera Ethiopian	1 piece, 28g	25	5.1	0.8	1	0.2
Bread Italian	1 slice, 28g	73	13.5	0.6	2.7	0.8
Bread Multi-Grain	1 slice, 28g	74	12.1	2.1	3.7	1.2
Bread Oat Bran	1 slice, 28g	66	11.1	1.3	2.9	1.2
Bread Oatmeal	1 slice, 28g	75	13.6	1.1	2.4	1.2
Bread Onion	1 slice, 28g	66	12.4	0.5	2.1	0.8

FOOD	SERVING SIZE	CALORIES	TOTAL CARB (g)	FIBER (g)	PROTEIN (g)	FAT (g)
Bread Paratha Whole Wheat	1 slice, 28g	91	12.7	2.7	1.8	3.7
Bread Pita	½ small , 28g	77	15.6	0.6	2.5	0.3
Bread Protein	1 slice, 28g	69	12.3	0.8	3.4	0.6
Bread Pumpernickel	1 slice, 28g	70	13.3	1.8	2.4	0.9
Bread Rice Bran	1 slice, 28g	68	12.2	1.4	2.5	1.3
Bread Rye	1 slice, 28g	73	13.5	3.4	2.4	0.9
Bread Rye	1 slice, 28g	73	13.5	1.6	2.4	0.9
Bread Rye Toasted	1 slice, 28g	80	14.9	1.8	2.6	1
Bread Soy	1 slice, 28g	72	11.8	1.2	4.3	1
Bread Wheat Sprouted	1 slice, 28g	53	9.5	1.5	3.7	0
Bread Whole Wheat	1 slice, 28g	61	11.9	3.1	3.7	0.8
Bread Whole Wheat	1 slice, 28g	69	13.3	1.9	2.6	1.1
Bread Whole Wheat	1 slice, 28g	71	12	1.7	3.5	1

FOOD	SERVING SIZE	CALORIES	TOTAL CARB (g)	FIBER (g)	PROTEIN (g)	FAT (g)
Cornbread Homemade	⅛ medium, 30g	85	12.8	0.5	1.9	2.8
Cornbread Muffin Homemade	1 small, 28g	85	12.8	0.4	1.9	2.8
Crackers Gluten-Free Multigrain/Multi-Seeded	3 crackers, 28g	127	18.6	2.9	3.2	4.4
Crackers Multigrain	4 crackers, 28g	135	18.9	1	2	5.7
Crackers Whole-Wheat	1 serving, 28g	120	19.5	2.9	3	4
Crumpet	1 small, 28g	54	8	0.5	2	1.6
Crumpet Toasted	1 small, 28g	61	8.9	0.5	2.3	1.7
Dumpling Plain	1 small, 28g	35	5.7	0.2	0.9	0.9
English Muffin Wheat Bran	1 muffin, 28g	65	13.5	1.3	2.3	0.5
English Muffin Whole Wheat	1 muffin, 28g	64	13.4	1.3	2.3	0.5
English Muffins	1 oz, 28g	62	12.5	1.3	2.4	0.6
English Muffins Mixed-Grain	1 oz, 28g	66	13	0.8	2.5	0.5
English Muffins Whole Grain White	1 muffin, 28g	69	14	1	2	0.5
English Muffins Whole-Wheat	1 oz, 28g	57	11.3	1.9	2.5	0.6

FOOD	SERVING SIZE	CALORIES	TOTAL CARB (g)	FIBER (g)	PROTEIN (g)	FAT (g)
French Toast	1 oz, 28g	60	9	0.3	2.1	1.7
Gluten-Free Crust Pizza with Cheese & Veggies, Thick	⅛ medium, 28g	64	7.4	0.8	1.8	3
Gluten-Free Crust Pizza with Cheese & Veggies, Thin	⅛ medium, 28g	62	6.2	0.7	1.9	3.4
Muffin English Cracked Wheat	1 muffin, 28g	64	13.4	1.3	2.3	0.5
Muffins Oat Bran	1 oz, 28g	76	13.5	1.3	2	2.1
Muffins Plain	1 oz, 28g	83	11.6	0.8	1.9	3.2
Multi-Grain Toast	1 oz, 28g	81	13.2	2.3	4.1	1.3
Naan Indian Flatbread	½ small , 28g	87	14.1	1.5	3.1	2
Pancakes Whole-Wheat Homemade	½ small , 28g	58	8.2	0.8	2.4	1.8
Pita Whole Wheat	⅛ medium, 28g	73	15.6	1.7	2.7	0.5
Pizza Extra Cheese, Thick Crust	⅛ medium, 28g	76	8.9	0.6	3.2	3.1
Pizza Extra Cheese, Thin Crust	⅛ medium, 28g	85	8.3	0.7	3.8	4
Pizza No Cheese, Thick Crust	⅛ medium, 28g	82	10.6	0.6	2.1	3.4

FOOD	SERVING SIZE	CALORIES	TOTAL CARB (g)	FIBER (g)	PROTEIN (g)	FAT (g)
Pizza No Cheese, Thin Crust	⅛ medium, 28g	77	8.6	0.6	2.1	3.8
Roll Cheese	1 roll, 28g	88	13.9	0.5	3.2	2.2
Roll Garlic	1 roll, 28g	87	14.5	0.6	3	1.8
Rolls Dinner Oat Bran	1 roll, 28g	66	11.3	1.1	2.7	1.3
Rolls Dinner Plain	1 roll, 28g	88	15	0.5	2.4	2
Rolls Dinner Rye	1 roll, 28g	80	14.9	1.4	2.9	1
Rolls Dinner Whole-Wheat	1 roll, 28g	74	14.3	2.1	2.4	1.3
Rolls Gluten-Free Brown Rice Flour/Tapioca Starch/Sorghum Flour	1 roll, 28g	72	11.3	0.8	1.6	2.3
Rolls Gluten-Free Whole Grain Tapioca Starch/Brown Rice Flour	1 roll, 28g	92	12.4	3.1	3.3	3.2
Rolls Hamburger Mixed-Grain	1 oz, 28g	74	12.5	1.1	2.7	1.7
Rolls Hamburger Plain	1 roll, 28g	78	14	0.5	2.7	1.1
Rolls Hamburger Wheat/cracked Wheat	1 roll, 28g	75	13.2	1.2	3.3	1
Rolls Hamburger Whole Grain	1 roll, 28g	71	13	0.6	2.6	1
Rolls Hamburger Whole Wheat	1 roll, 28g	75	12.6	1.7	3.5	1.2
Rolls Hard	1 roll, 28g	82	14.8	0.6	2.8	1.2

FOOD	SERVING SIZE	CALORIES	TOTAL CARB (g)	FIBER (g)	PROTEIN (g)	FAT (g)
Rolls Pumpernickel	1 roll, 28g	77	14.5	1.5	3	0.8
Thick Crust Gluten-Free Cheese Pizza	⅛ medium, 28g	73	8.4	0.8	2.1	3.4
Thick Crust Whole Wheat Cheese Pizza	⅛ medium, 28g	76	9.4	1.3	3	3.2
Thin Crust Gluten-Free Cheese Pizza	⅛ medium, 28g	74	7.2	0.7	2.3	4
Thin Crust Whole Wheat Cheese Pizza	⅛ medium, 28g	76	8.1	1.1	3.1	3.7
Tortilla	1 medium, 30g	79	14.1	1.5	2.1	1.6
Whole Wheat Crust Pizza with Cheese & Veggies, Thick	⅛ medium, 28g	66	8.2	1.1	2.5	2.8
Whole Wheat Crust Pizza with Cheese & Veggies, Thin	⅛ medium, 28g	65	6.9	1	2.5	3.2
Wonton Wrappers	1 oz, 28g	81	16.2	0.5	2.7	0.4

3
BEANS AND PULSES

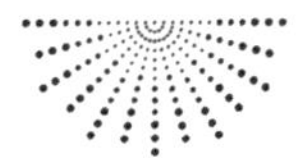

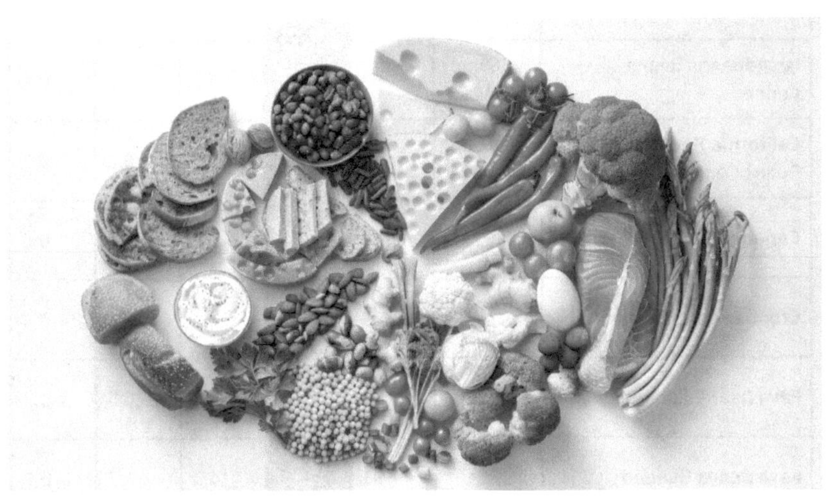

FOOD	SERVING SIZE	CALORIES	TOTAL CARB (g)	FIBER (g)	PROTEIN (g)	FAT (g)
Adzuki Beans Cooked	½ cup, 115 g	147	28.5	8.4	8.6	0.1
Baked Beans Canned	½ cup, 127 g	133	26	7	6.1	0.5
Black Beans Cooked	½ cup, 86 g	114	20.4	7.5	7.6	0.5
Black Turtle Beans Canned	½ cup, 120 g	109	19.9	8.3	7.2	0.3
Black Turtle Beans Cooked	½ cup, 93 g	121	22.6	7.7	7.6	0.3
Broadbeans Cooked	½ cup, 85 g	94	16.7	4.6	6.5	0.3
Broadbeans Beans Canned	½ cup, 128 g	91	15.9	4.7	7	0.3
California Red Kidney Beans Cooked	½ cup, 89 g	110	19.9	8.3	8.1	0.1
Catjang Beans Cooked	½ cup, 89 g	104	18.1	3.2	7.2	0.6
Cranberry Beans Canned	½ cup, 130 g	108	19.7	8.2	7.2	0.4
Fava Beans Cooked	½ cup, 85 g	94	16.7	4.6	6.5	0.3
Fava Beans Canned	½ cup, 128 g	91	15.9	4.7	7	0.3
French Beans Cooked	½ cup, 89 g	115	21.4	8.4	6.3	0.7

FOOD	SERVING SIZE	CALORIES	TOTAL CARB (g)	FIBER (g)	PROTEIN (g)	FAT (g)
Great Northern Beans Canned	½ cup, 131 g	149	27.5	6.4	9.7	0.5
Great Northern Beans Cooked	½ cup, 89 g	105	18.8	6.2	7.4	0.4
Green Beans Canned	½ cup, 120 g	18	3.9	1.8	0.9	0.2
Green Beans Cooked	½ cup, 68 g	19	4.4	2	1	0.1
Green Snap Beans Cooked	½ cup, 63 g	22	5	2	1.2	0.2
Hyacinth Beans Beans Cooked	½ cup, 97 g	113	20.1	0	7.9	0.6
Hyacinth-Beans Immature Seeds Drained	½ cup, 44 g	22	4	0	1.3	0.1
Kidney Bean Sprouts	½ cup, 92 g	27	3.8	0	3.9	0.5
Kidney Beans Canned	½ cup, 128 g	108	18.6	5.5	6.7	0.8
Kidney Beans Cooked	½ cup, 89 g	113	20.3	5.7	7.7	0.4
Kidney Red Beans Canned	½ cup, 128 g	104	19	6.8	6.7	0.5
Large White Beans Cooked	½ cup, 90 g	125	22.6	5.7	8.8	0.3
Lima Baby Beans	½ cup, 91 g	115	21.2	7	7.3	0.3
Lima Beans Canned	½ cup, 124 g	88	16.5	4.5	5	0.4

FOOD	SERVING SIZE	CALORIES	TOTAL CARB (g)	FIBER (g)	PROTEIN (g)	FAT (g)
Lima Beans Cooked	½ cup, 85 g	105	20.1	4.6	5.8	0.3
Lima Beans Immature Seeds Boiled	½ cup, 90 g	95	17.5	4.3	6	0.3
Lima Beans Immature Seeds Canned	½ cup, 124 g	88	16.5	4.5	5	0.4
Lima Beans Immature Seeds Cooked	½ cup, 90 g	92	17.3	4.8	5.4	0.3
Mothbeans Beans	½ cup, 89 g	104	18.7	0	7	0.5
Mung Bean Sprouts Boiled	½ cup, 52 g	16	3.1	0.9	1.6	0.1
Mung Bean Sprouts Canned	½ cup, 63 g	8	1.3	0.5	0.9	0
Mung Beans Cooked	½ cup, 101 g	106	19.3	7.7	7.1	0.4
Mungo Beans Cooked	½ cup, 90 g	95	16.5	5.8	6.8	0.5
Navy Beans Canned	½ cup, 131 g	148	26.8	6.7	9.9	0.6
Navy Beans Cooked	½ cup, 91 g	127	23.7	9.6	7.5	0.6
Pink Beans Canned	½ cup, 90 g	133	24.9	4.8	8.1	0.4
Pink Beans Cooked	½ cup, 90 g	133	25	4.8	8.1	0.4
Pinto Beans Canned	½ cup, 139 g	158	28.1	7.6	9.7	1.3

FOOD	SERVING SIZE	CALORIES	TOTAL CARB (g)	FIBER (g)	PROTEIN (g)	FAT (g)
Pinto Beans Cooked	½ cup, 86 g	123	22.5	7.7	7.7	0.6
Red Kidney Beans Cooked	½ cup, 89 g	113	20.3	6.6	7.7	0.4
Red Mexican Beans Canned	½ cup, 90 g	123	22.7	6.9	6.9	0.8
Red Mexican Beans Cooked	½ cup, 90 g	128	23.5	8	8.1	0.6
Roman Beans	½ cup, 89 g	121	21.8	7.7	8.3	0.4
Shellie Beans Canned	½ cup, 123 g	37	7.6	4.2	2.2	0.2
Small White Beans Cooked	½ cup, 90 g	128	23.2	9.4	8.1	0.6
Snap Beans Green All Styles	½ cup, 56 g	18	3.9	1.9	1.1	0.2
Snap Green Canned	½ cup, 77 g	17	3.3	1.5	0.9	0.4
Snap Yellow Canned	½ cup, 77 g	15	3.5	1	0.9	0.1
Soybeans (Edamame) Boiled	½ cup, 86 g	148	7.2	5.2	15.7	7.7
String Green Beans Cooked	½ cup, 63 g	22	4.9	2	1.2	0.2
String Yellow Beans Cooked	½ cup, 63 g	22	4.9	2.1	1.2	0.2
White Beans Canned	½ cup, 131 g	149	27.8	6.3	9.5	0.4

FOOD	SERVING SIZE	CALORIES	TOTAL CARB (g)	FIBER (g)	PROTEIN (g)	FAT (g)
White Beans Cooked	½ cup, 90 g	124	22.5	5.7	8.7	0.3
White Lima Beans Canned	½ cup, 121 g	96	18	5.8	6	0.2
Yardlong Beans Boiled	½ cup, 86 g	101	18.1	3.3	7.1	0.4
Yellow Beans Cooked	½ cup, 89 g	128	22.5	9.3	8.2	1
Yellow Snap Beans Cooked	½ cup, 63 g	22	5	2.1	1.2	0.2

4

BEEF, VEAL, LAMB, PORK, POULTRY

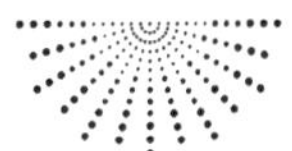

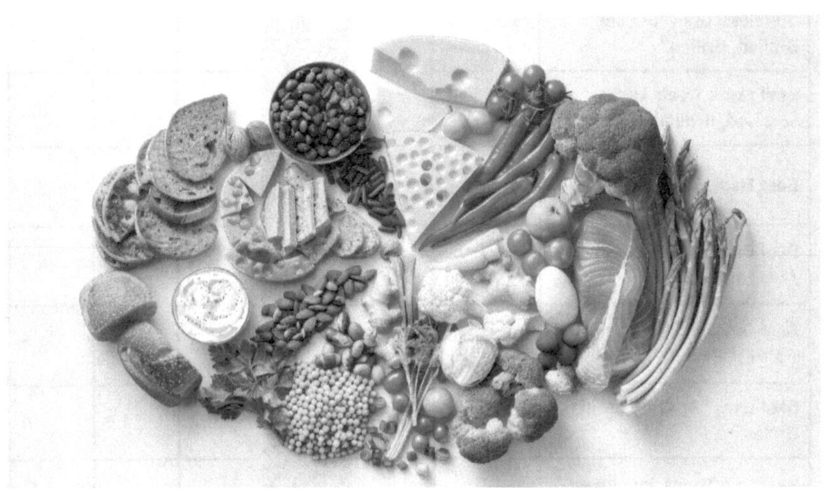

FOOD	SERVING SIZE	CALORIES	TOTAL CARB (g)	FIBER (g)	PROTEIN (g)	FAT (g)
Beef Brisket Lean, "Braised, Broiled, Grilled"	3 oz, 85g	184	0	0	25.1	8.5
Beef Brisket Flat Half, Boneless, Lean, "Braised, Broiled, Grilled"	3 oz, 85g	180	0	0	27.7	6.9
Beef Brisket Flat Half, Boneless, Lean Raw	4 oz, 114g	156	0	0	24.3	6.6
Beef Chuck Clod Roast Lean "Braised, Broiled, Grilled"	3 oz, 85g	145	0	0	22.1	5.7
Beef Chuck Eye Roast Lean Raw	4 oz, 114g	159	0	0	23.6	7.1
Beef Chuck Eye Roast Boneless Lean "Braised, Broiled, Grilled"	3 oz, 85g	162	0	0	22.4	8
Beef Flank Steak Lean "Braised, Broiled, Grilled"	3 oz, 85g	151	0	0	23.8	5.5
Beef Flank Steak Lean Raw	4 oz, 114g	170	0	0	24.8	7.2
Beef Ground 95% Lean Meat / 5% Fat Raw	4 oz, 114g	156	0	0	24.4	5.7
Beef Ground 97% Lean Meat / 3% Fat Raw	4 oz, 114g	138	0	0	25.1	3.4
Beef Liver "Braised, Broiled, Grilled"	3 oz, 85g	161	4.3	0.2	24.5	4.4
Beef Loin Tenderloin Roast Boneless Lean Raw	4 oz, 114g	163	0	0	24.8	7
Beef Loin Tenderloin Roast Boneless Lean "Braised, Broiled, Grilled"	3 oz, 85g	156	0	0	23.4	6.9

FOOD	SERVING SIZE	CALORIES	TOTAL CARB (g)	FIBER (g)	PROTEIN (g)	FAT (g)
Beef Loin Tenderloin Steak Boneless Lean "Braised, Broiled, Grilled"	3 oz, 85g	179	0	0	25.9	7.7
Beef Loin Tenderloin Steak Boneless Lean Raw	4 oz, 114g	163	0	0	24.8	7
Beef Loin Top Sirloin Petite Roast Boneless Lean "Braised, Broiled, Grilled"	3 oz, 85g	147	0	0	24.6	5.4
Beef Loin Top Sirloin Petite Roast/filet Boneless Lean Raw	4 oz, 114g	151	0	0	26.3	5
Beef Plate Steak Boneless Inside Skirt Lean Raw	4 oz, 114g	195	0	0	23.8	11.1
Beef Ribeye Petite Roast/filet Boneless Lean Raw	4 oz, 114g	157	0.2	0	25.7	6
Beef Ribeye Cap Steak Boneless Lean Raw	4 oz, 114g	193	1.3	0.1	22.9	10.7
Beef Ribeye Filet Boneless Lean "Braised, Broiled, Grilled"	3 oz, 85g	169	0.1	0	24.5	7.8
Beef Ribeye Petite Roast Boneless Lean "Braised, Broiled, Grilled"	3 oz, 85g	160	0	0	23.8	7.2
Beef Roast Lean "Braised, Broiled, Grilled"	3 oz, 85g	128	0	0	24.8	3.2
Beef Round Bottom Round Steak Lean, "Braised, Broiled, Grilled"	3 oz, 85g	190	0	0	28.1	7.7
Beef Round Eye Of Round Roast Boneless Lean Raw	3 oz, 85g	105	0	0	19.8	2.9

FOOD	SERVING SIZE	CALORIES	TOTAL CARB (g)	FIBER (g)	PROTEIN (g)	FAT (g)
Beef Round Eye Of Round Roast Boneless Lean "Braised, Broiled, Grilled"/Grilled	3 oz, 85g	141	0	0	25.4	3.6
Beef Round Eye Of Round Steak Boneless Lean Raw	4 oz, 114g	141	0	0	26.6	3.9
Beef Short Loin Porterhouse Steak Lean "Braised, Broiled, Grilled"	3 oz, 85g	165	0	0	22.9	7.5
Beef Shoulder Pot Roast Boneless Lean "Braised, Broiled, Grilled"	3 oz, 85g	170	0	0	26.6	7.1
Beef Shoulder Pot Roast or Steak Boneless Lean Raw	4 oz, 114g	143	0.1	0	24.5	5
Beef Shoulder Steak Boneless Lean "Braised, Broiled, Grilled"	3 oz, 85g	151	0	0	24.3	5.3
Beef Shoulder Top Blade Steak Boneless Lean "Braised, Broiled, Grilled"	3 oz, 85g	172	0	0	24	8.4
Beef Shoulder Top Blade Steak Boneless Lean Raw	4 oz, 114g	163	0	0	23.2	7.8
Beef Top Sirloin Steak Lean "Braised, Broiled, Grilled"	3 oz, 85g	160	0	0	25.7	5.6
Beef Tri-Tip Roast, Bottom Sirloin, 0 Inch Fat, Lean Raw	4 oz, 114g	162	0	0	24.2	6.4
Beef Tri-Tip Roast, Bottom Sirloin, Lean, Lean "Braised, Broiled, Grilled"	3 oz, 85g	164	0	0	22.4	8.3
Chicken Breast Lean "Braised, Broiled, Grilled"	3 oz, 85g	134	0	0	27.3	2.8

FOOD	SERVING SIZE	CALORIES	TOTAL CARB (g)	FIBER (g)	PROTEIN (g)	FAT (g)
Chicken Breast Raw	4 oz, 114g	137	0	0	25.7	3
Chicken Capons Giblets Raw	1 giblets, 115g	150	1.6	0.1	21	6
Chicken Drumstick Skinless Raw	4 oz, 114g	132	0	0	22.1	4.2
Chicken Drumsticks Raw	4 oz, 114g	184	0.1	0	20.6	10.5
Chicken Fillet Grilled	3 oz, 85g	123	2	0	18.9	4.4
Chicken Gizzard All Classes Raw	4 oz, 114g	107	0	0	20.1	2.3
Chicken Ground Raw	4 oz, 114g	163	0	0	19.9	9.2
Chicken Leg Boneless Skinless Raw	4 oz, 114g	137	0	0	21.8	4.8
Chicken Wing Broiler	2 wing, 102g	190	0.6	0	28.9	7.9
Cornish Game Hen Skinless, "Braised, Broiled, Grilled"	3 oz, 85g	113	0	0	19.6	3.3
Duck Domesticated Meat Only Raw	4 oz, 114g	154	1.1	0	20.8	6.8
Duck Wild Breast Meat Only Raw	4 oz, 114g	140	0	0	22.6	4.8
Egg Duck Boiled/Poached	1 egg, 70g	146	1.1	0	10.1	10.9
Egg Duck Whole Raw	1 egg, 70g	130	1	0	9	9.6

FOOD	SERVING SIZE	CALORIES	TOTAL CARB (g)	FIBER (g)	PROTEIN (g)	FAT (g)
Egg Goose Boiled/Poached	½ egg, 72g	150	1.1	0	11.3	10.8
Egg Goose Whole Raw	½ egg, 72g	133	1	0	10	9.6
Egg Quail Whole Raw	1 egg, 9g	14	0	0	1.2	1
Egg Turkey Whole Raw	1 egg, 79g	135	0.9	0	10.8	9.4
Egg White Boiled/Poached	1 large, 24g	14	0.2	0	2.9	0
Egg White Raw	1 large, 33g	17	0.2	0	3.6	0.1
Egg Whole Boiled/Poached	1 small, 37g	53	0.3	0	4.6	3.5
Egg Yolks Raw	1 large, 17g	55	0.6	0	2.7	4.5
Goat Ribs Cooked	2 rib, 92g	131	0	0	24.7	2.8
Goose Domesticated Meat Only Raw	4 oz, 114g	184	0	0	25.9	8.1
Lamb Loin Chop Lean "Braised, Broiled, Grilled"	3 oz, 85g	182	0	0	25.3	8.2
Lamb Roast Lean "Braised, Broiled, Grilled"	3 oz, 85g	167	0	0	22.4	7.8
Pheasant Meat Only Raw	4 oz, 114g	152	0	0	26.9	4.1
Pork Chops Lean	3 oz, 85g	166	0	0	26.4	5.9
Pork Enhanced Loin Tenderloin Lean Raw	4 oz, 114g	121	0	0	23.2	2.4

FOOD	SERVING SIZE	CALORIES	TOTAL CARB (g)	FIBER (g)	PROTEIN (g)	FAT (g)
Pork Fresh Leg Rump Half Lean "Braised, Broiled, Grilled"	3 oz, 85g	140	0	0	24.5	3.9
Pork Ground 96% Lean & 4% Fat Raw	4 oz, 114g	138	0.2	0	24.1	4.6
Pork Leg Rump Half Lean Raw	4 oz, 114g	137	0	0	24.9	3.3
Pork Leg Shank Half Lean Raw	4 oz, 114g	136	0	0	24.7	3.4
Pork Leg Shank Half Lean "Braised, Broiled, Grilled"	3 oz, 85g	149	0	0	24.4	5
Pork Leg Whole Lean Raw	4 oz, 114g	155	0	0	23.3	6.2
Pork Loin Backribs Bone-In Lean Raw	4 oz, 114g	196	0	0	23.8	11.2
Pork Loin Blade (Chops Or Roasts) Boneless Lean Raw	4 oz, 114g	140	0.9	0	24.3	4.3
Pork Loin Blade Bone-In Lean Raw	4 oz, 114g	163	0	0	24.2	6.7
Pork Loin Center Rib Bone-In Lean "Braised, Broiled, Grilled"	3 oz, 85g	158	0	0	21.9	7.1
Pork Loin Center Rib Bone-In Lean Raw	4 oz, 114g	155	0	0	24.8	5.5
Pork Loin Center Rib Bone-In Separable Lean "Braised, Broiled, Grilled"	3 oz, 85g	177	0	0	24.7	7.9
Pork Loin Center Rib Boneless Lean Raw	4 oz, 114g	173	0	0	24.9	7.4

FOOD	SERVING SIZE	CALORIES	TOTAL CARB (g)	FIBER (g)	PROTEIN (g)	FAT (g)
Pork Loin Country-Style Ribs Lean Raw	4 oz, 114g	160	0	0	23.7	6.4
Pork Loin Tenderloin Lean "Braised, Broiled, Grilled"	3 oz, 85g	159	0	0	25.9	5.4
Pork Loin Tenderloin Lean Raw	4 oz, 114g	124	0	0	23.9	2.5
Pork Loin Top Loin Boneless Lean Raw	4 oz, 114g	145	0	0	25.5	3.9
Pork Loin Top Loin Boneless Lean "Braised, Broiled, Grilled"	3 oz, 85g	147	0	0	23.1	5.3
Pork Shoulder Whole Lean Raw	4 oz, 114g	169	0	0	22.3	8.1
Pork Steak/Cutlet Broiled/Baked Lean	3 oz, 85g	145	0.1	0	20.9	6.3
Pork Tenderloin Baked	3 oz, 85g	131	0	0	22.9	3.7
Pork Tenderloin Lean "Braised, Broiled, Grilled"	3 oz, 85g	121	0	0	23.2	2.4
Tripe Cooked	3 oz, 85g	76	0	0	10.7	3.3
Turkey Back Meat Only Raw	4 oz, 114g	129	0.2	0	24.3	2.9
Turkey Back Meat Only Roasted	3 oz, 85g	147	0	0	23.6	5.1
Turkey Breast Meat Only Raw	4 oz, 114g	130	0.2	0	27	1.7
Turkey Dark Meat Skin not Eaten Roasted	3 oz, 85g	142	0	0	22.9	5.1

FOOD	SERVING SIZE	CALORIES	TOTAL CARB (g)	FIBER (g)	PROTEIN (g)	FAT (g)
Turkey Drumstick Cooked Skinless	3 oz, 85g	122	0	0	24.2	2.9
Turkey Drumstick Raw	4 oz, 114g	124	0.2	0	27	1.7
Turkey Drumstick Roasted Skinless	3 oz, 85g	122	0	0	24.2	2.9
Turkey Ground Raw Fatfree	1 patty raw, 114g	128	0	0	26.9	2.2
Turkey Sausage Fresh Raw	4 oz, 114g	177	0.5	0	21.4	9.2
Turkey Whole Giblets Raw	4 oz, 114g	141	0.1	0	20.7	5.8
Turkey Whole Meat Raw	4 oz, 114g	131	0.2	0	25.8	2.2
Veal Chop Lean Cooked 'Braised/Broiled/Grilled"	5.75 oz Raw, 85g	148	0	0	22.2	5.8
Veal Cutlet/Steak Lean "Braised, Broiled, Grilled"	3 oz, 85g	154	0	0	28	3.9
Veal Foreshank Lean "Braised, Broiled, Grilled"	3 oz, 85g	134	0	0	24.8	3.8
Veal Leg (Top Round) Lean Raw	4 oz, 114g	122	0	0	24.3	2
Veal Loin Chop Lean "Braised, Broiled, Grilled"	3 oz, 85g	135	0.1	0	25.3	3.8
Veal Loin Lean "Braised, Broiled, Grilled"	3 oz, 85g	192	0	0	28.5	7.8
Veal Loin Lean Raw	4 oz, 114g	130	0	0	24.9	3.3

FOOD	SERVING SIZE	CALORIES	TOTAL CARB (g)	FIBER (g)	PROTEIN (g)	FAT (g)
Veal Rib Lean "Braised, Broiled, Grilled"	3 oz, 85g	185	0	0	29.3	6.6
Veal Shank Lean Raw	4 oz, 114g	107	0	0	22.5	1.9
Veal Shoulder Arm Lean "Braised, Broiled, Grilled"	3 oz, 85g	171	0	0	30.4	4.5
Veal Shoulder Arm Lean Raw	4 oz, 114g	120	0	0	22.8	2.5
Veal Sirloin Lean "Braised, Broiled, Grilled"	3 oz, 85g	173	0	0	28.9	5.5
Veal Sirloin Lean Raw	4 oz, 114g	125	0	0	23	3
Veal Top Round Lean "Braised, Broiled, Grilled"	3 oz, 85g	128	0	0	23.9	2.9

5

DAIRY AND PLANT-BASED ALTERNATIVES

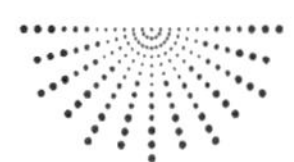

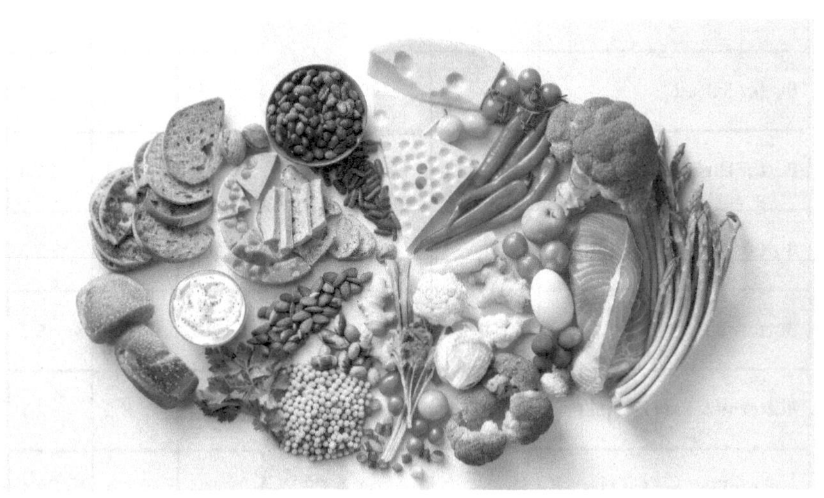

FOOD	SERVING SIZE	CALORIES	TOTAL CARB (g)	SODIUM (mg)	PROTEIN (g)	FAT (g)
Almond Milk Unsweetened	1 cup, 244g	37	1.4	173	1.4	2.7
American Cheese	1 slice, 28g	92	2.4	360	4.7	7.2
American Cheese Spread	1 tbsp, 15g	44	1.3	244	2.5	3.2
Blue Cheese	1 oz, 28.4g	100	0.7	325	6.1	8.2
Brick Cheese	1 oz, 28.4g	105	0.8	159	6.6	8.4
Brie Cheese	1 oz, 28.4g	95	0.1	179	5.9	7.9
Butter Salted	1 tbsp, 14g	100	0	90	0.1	11.4
Butter Unsalted	1 tbsp, 14g	100	0	2	0.1	11.4
Butter Whipped Salted	1 tbsp, 3g	22	0	17	0	2.3
Buttermilk	1 cup, 245g	152	12	257	7.9	8.1
Buttermilk Fat Free (Skim)	1 cup, 244g	98	11.7	464	8.1	2.1
Buttermilk Low Fat (1%)	1 cup, 244g	98	11.7	464	8.1	2.1
Camembert	1 oz, 28.4g	85	0.1	239	5.6	6.9

FOOD	SERVING SIZE	CALORIES	TOTAL CARB (g)	SODIUM (mg)	PROTEIN (g)	FAT (g)
Caraway Cheese	1 oz, 28.4g	107	0.9	196	7.2	8.3
Cheddar Cheese Reduced Fat	1 slice, 21g	66	0.6	132	5.7	4.3
Cheddar Cheese	1 oz, 28.4g	115	0.9	185	6.5	9.5
Cheese Cream Low Fat	1 oz, 28.4g	59	1.9	90	2.2	4.7
Cheese Dry White Queso Seco	1 oz, 28.4g	92	0.6	513	7	6.9
Colby Cheese	1 oz, 28.4g	112	0.7	172	6.7	9.1
Colby Jack Cheese	1 oz, 28.4g	109	0.5	171	6.9	8.9
Cottage Cheese (Blended)	1 cup, 226g	221	7.6	712	25.1	9.7
Cottage Cheese 1% fat No Added Sodium	1 cup, 226g	163	6.1	29	28	2.3
Cottage Cheese Low-fat With Fruit	1 cup, 226g	160	18.7	452	15.5	3.3
Cottage Cheese Nonfat	1 cup, 226g	163	15.1	841	23.4	0.7
Cream Cheese	1 tbsp, 14.5g	51	0.8	46	0.9	5
Cream Half and Half	1 tbsp, 15g	20	0.6	9	0.5	1.7
Cream Half and Half Fat Free	1 tbsp, 15g	9	1.4	15	0.4	0.2

FOOD	SERVING SIZE	CALORIES	TOTAL CARB (g)	SODIUM (mg)	PROTEIN (g)	FAT (g)
Cream Half and Half Low-fat	1 tbsp, 15g	11	0.5	8	0.5	0.8
Cream Heavy Whipping	1 tbsp, 15g	51	0.4	4	0.4	5.4
Cultured Sour Cream	1 tbsp, 12g	24	0.6	4	0.3	2.3
Dried Whey Powder (Acid)	1 oz, 30g	102	22	290	3.5	0.2
Edam Cheese	1 oz, 28.4g	101	0.4	276	7.1	8.1
Feta Cheese	1 oz, 28.4g	75	1.1	323	4	6.1
Fontina Cheese	1 oz, 28.4g	110	0.4	227	7.3	8.8
Ghee -Clarified Butter	1 tbsp, 12.8g	112	0	0	0	12.7
Gjetost Cheese	1 oz, 28.4g	132	12.1	170	2.7	8.4
Goat Cheese	1 oz, 28.4g	102	0.2	123	6.7	8.2
Goat Cheese Hard	1 oz, 28.4g	128	0.6	120	8.7	10.1
Goat Cheese Soft	1 oz, 28.4g	75	0	130	5.3	6
Goat Milk	1 oz, 30.5g	21	1.4	15	1.1	1.3
Gouda Cheese	1 oz, 28.4g	101	0.6	233	7.1	7.8

FOOD	SERVING SIZE	CALORIES	TOTAL CARB (g)	SODIUM (mg)	PROTEIN (g)	FAT (g)
Grated Parmesan	1 tbsp, 5g	21	0.7	90	1.4	1.4
Grated Parmesan Cheese (Low-Sodium)	1 tbsp, 5g	23	0.2	3	2.1	1.5
Gruyere Cheese	1 oz, 28.4g	117	0.1	203	8.5	9.2
Kefir Low-fat Plain	1 cup, 245g	105	11.7	98	9.3	2.5
Light Cream - Coffee Cream	1 tbsp, 15g	29	0.5	11	0.4	2.9
Light Whipping Cream	1 tbsp, 15g	44	0.4	5	0.3	4.6
Limburger Cheese	1 oz, 28.4g	93	0.1	227	5.7	7.7
Mexican Cheese Blend Low Fat	1 oz, 28.4g	80	1	220	7	5.5
Mexican Cheese Queso Anejo	1 oz, 28.4g	106	1.3	321	6.1	8.5
Milk Buttermilk Dried	¼ cup, 30g	116	14.7	155	10.3	1.7
Milk Buttermilk Fluid Cultured	1 cup, 245g	137	13	257	10	4.9
Milk Dehydrated	¼ cup, 32g	159	12.3	119	8.4	8.5
Milk Evaporated	1 cup, 252g	197	28.6	290	19	0.5
Milk High Fat (3.7% Fat)	1 cup, 244g	156	11.3	120	8	8.9

FOOD	SERVING SIZE	CALORIES	TOTAL CARB (g)	SODIUM (mg)	PROTEIN (g)	FAT (g)
Milk Indian Buffalo Fluid	1 cup, 244g	237	12.6	127	9.2	16.8
Milk Non-Dairy	1 cup, 244g	78	9.6	142	2.7	3.1
Milk Sheep Fluid	1 cup, 245g	265	13.1	108	14.7	17.2
Milk Skim	1 cup, 245g	83	12.2	103	8.3	0.2
Milk Whole	1 cup, 244g	149	11.7	105	7.7	7.9
Monterey Cheese	1 oz, 28.4g	106	0.2	170	7	8.6
Monterey Cheese Low Fat	1 oz, 28.4g	89	0.2	222	8	6.1
Mozzarella	1 oz, 28.4g	85	0.7	138	6.3	6.3
Mozzarella Cheese Fat Free	1 oz, 28.4g	40	1	211	9	0
Mozzarella Low-fat	1 oz, 28.4g	72	0.8	176	6.9	4.5
Muenster Cheese	1 oz, 28.4g	105	0.3	178	6.6	8.5
Muenster Cheese Low Fat	1 oz, 28.4g	77	1	170	7	5
Neufchatel Cheese	1 oz, 28.4g	72	1	95	2.6	6.5
Parmesan Cheese Dry Low Fat	⅔ cup, 150g	398	2.1	2294	30	30

FOOD	SERVING SIZE	CALORIES	TOTAL CARB (g)	SODIUM (mg)	PROTEIN (g)	FAT (g)
Port De Salut Cheese	1 oz, 28.4g	100	0.2	152	6.8	8
Provolone Cheese	1 oz, 28.4g	100	0.6	206	7.3	7.6
Puerto Rican White Cheese	1 oz, 28.4g	49	0.9	24	3.2	3.7
Queso Asadero	1 oz, 28.4g	101	0.8	200	6.4	8
Queso Blanco	1 oz, 28.4g	88	0.7	200	5.8	6.9
Queso Chihuahua	1 oz, 28.4g	106	1.6	175	6.1	8.4
Queso Cotija	1 oz, 28.4g	104	1.1	398	5.7	8.5
Queso Fresco	1 oz, 28.4g	85	0.8	213	5.1	6.8
Ricotta Cheese	½ cup, 124g	193	5.1	114	14	12.9
Romano Cheese	1 tbsp, 5g	19	0.2	72	1.6	1.3
Roquefort	1 oz, 28.4g	105	0.6	514	6.1	8.7
Sharp Cheddar Cheese	1 oz, 28.4g	116	0.6	183	6.9	9.6
Shredded Parmesan	1 tbsp, 5g	21	0.2	85	1.9	1.4
Spread Cream Cheese Base	1 tbsp, 14.5g	43	0.5	63	1	4.1

FOOD	SERVING SIZE	CALORIES	TOTAL CARB (g)	SODIUM (mg)	PROTEIN (g)	FAT (g)
Swiss Cheese	1 oz, 28.4g	112	0.4	53	7.7	8.8
Swiss Cheese Low Fat	1 oz, 28.4g	51	1	57	8.1	1.4
Swiss Cheese Low Sodium	1 oz, 28.4g	106	1	4	8.1	7.8
Tilsit Cheese	1 oz, 28.4g	97	0.5	214	6.9	7.4
Whey Acid Fluid	1 cup, 246g	59	12.6	118	1.9	0.2
Whey Fluid Sweet	1 cup, 246g	66	12.6	133	2.1	0.9
Whey Powder Dried Sweet	1 oz, 30g	106	22.3	324	3.9	0.3
Whipped Cream	2 tbsp, 60g	154	7.5	5	1.9	13.3
Yogurt Coconut Milk	6 oz, 170g	109	13.5	36	0.5	6
Yogurt Greek Fruit Whole Milk	⅔ cup, 150g	159	18.4	56	11	4.5
Yogurt Greek Low Fat Milk Fruit	⅔ cup, 150g	155	17.8	50	12.3	3.9
Yogurt Greek Nonfat	6 oz, 170g	100	6.1	61	17.3	0.7
Yogurt Greek Plain	⅔ cup, 150g	146	6	53	13.5	7.5
Yogurt Greek Whole Milk Natural Flavoring	⅔ cup, 150g	167	14	59	12.7	6.7

FOOD	SERVING SIZE	CALORIES	TOTAL CARB (g)	SODIUM (mg)	PROTEIN (g)	FAT (g)
Yogurt Greek With Oats	⅔ cup, 150g	231	35.7	125	13	4.7
Yogurt Liquid	1 cup, 240g	173	28.3	127	8.9	2.6
Yogurt Non-Fat	1 cup, 245g	137	18.8	189	14	0.4
Yogurt Plain	1 cup, 245g	149	11.4	113	8.5	8
Yogurt Whole Milk Fruit	⅔ cup, 150g	131	18.5	66	4.7	4.3
Yogurt Whole Milk Natural Flavoring	⅔ cup, 150g	116	14.1	66	5	4.6

6

FRUITS & FRUIT PRODUCTS

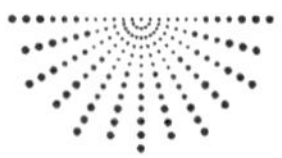

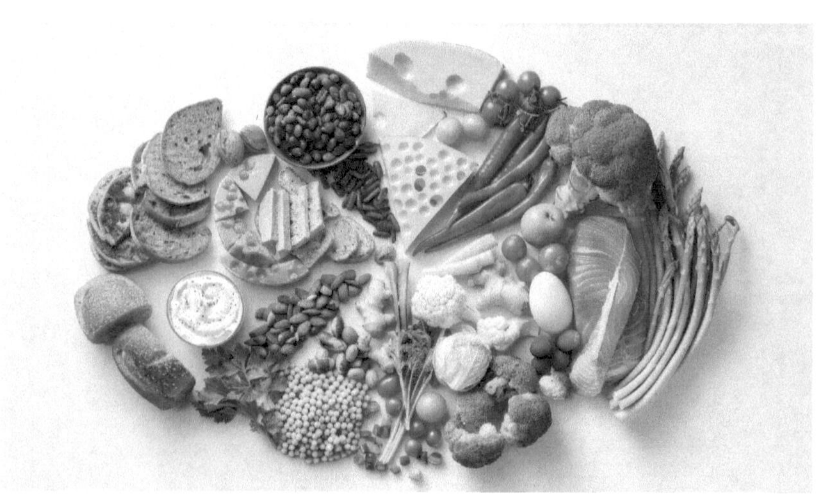

FOOD	SERVING SIZE	CALORIES	TOTAL CARB (g)	FIBER (g)	PROTEIN (g)	FAT (g)
Abiyuch	½ cup, 114g	79	20.1	6	1.7	0.1
Acerola Cherries	1 cup, 98g	31	7.5	1.1	0.4	0.3
Acerola Juice Raw	½ cup, 121g	28	5.8	0.4	0.5	0.4
Ambrosia	1 cup, 193g	135	31.2	4.4	1.7	1.9
Apple Baked Unsweetened	1 small, 101g	57	15	2.6	0.3	0.2
Apple Chips	¼ cup, 7g	32	5.2	0.7	0.1	1.5
Apple Juice	½ cup, 124g	57	14	0.2	0.1	0.2
Apples All Types	1 cup, 125g	65	17.3	3	0.3	0.2
Apples Fuji	1 cup, 109g	69	16.6	2.3	0.2	0.2
Apples Gala	1 cup, 109g	62	14.9	2.5	0.3	0.1
Apples Golden Delicious	1 cup, 109g	62	14.8	2.6	0.3	0.2
Apples Granny Smith	1 cup, 109g	63	14.8	3.1	0.5	0.2
Apples Red Delicious	1 cup, 109g	64	15.3	2.5	0.3	0.2
Apricot Nectar Canned	1 cup, 251g	141	34.2	0.3	0.4	1.1
Apricots	1 cup, 155g	74	17.2	3.1	2.2	0.6
Apricots Dried	¼ cup, 33g	80	20.7	2.4	1.1	0.2

FOOD	SERVING SIZE	CALORIES	TOTAL CARB (g)	FIBER (g)	PROTEIN (g)	FAT (g)
Apricots Light Syrup Pack	1 cup, 253g	159	41.7	4	1.3	0.1
Apricots Water-Packed	1 cup, 243g	66	15.5	3.9	1.7	0.4
Asian Pears	1 item, 122g	51	13	4.4	0.6	0.3
Avocados	1 cup, 150g	240	12.8	10.1	3	22
Avocados California	1 cup, 230g	384	19.9	15.6	4.5	35.4
Avocados Florida	1 cup, 230g	276	18	12.9	5.1	23.1
Banana Baked	1 small, 101g	128	32.9	2.9	1.2	0.4
Bananas	1 small, 101g	90	23.1	2.6	1.1	0.3
Bananas Dried	¼ cup, 25g	87	22.1	2.5	1	0.5
Black Currants European	1 cup, 112g	71	17.2	0	1.6	0.5
Blackberries	1 cup, 144g	62	13.8	7.6	2	0.7
Blackberry Juice Canned	½ cup, 125g	48	9.8	0.1	0.4	0.8
Blueberries	1 cup, 148g	84	21.4	3.6	1.1	0.5
Blueberries Water-Packed	1 cup, 244g	93	23.7	3.9	1.2	0.5
Boysenberries	1 cup, 132g	66	16.1	7	1.5	0.3
Breadfruit	1 cup, 220g	227	59.7	10.8	2.4	0.5

FOOD	SERVING SIZE	CALORIES	TOTAL CARB (g)	FIBER (g)	PROTEIN (g)	FAT (g)
Carissa	1 cup, 150g	93	20.4	0	0.8	2
Cherimoya	1 cup, 160g	120	28.3	4.8	2.5	1.1
Cherries Sour Red	1 cup, 155g	78	18.9	2.5	1.6	0.5
Cherries Sour Red Light Syrup Pack	1 cup, 252g	189	48.6	2	1.9	0.3
Cherries Sour Water-Packed	1 cup, 168g	71	17.6	2	1.2	0.4
Cherries Sweet	1 cup, 138g	87	22.1	2.9	1.5	0.3
Cherries Sweet Water-Packed	1 cup, 248g	114	29.2	3.7	1.9	0.3
Clementines	1 fruit, 74g	35	8.9	1.3	0.6	0.1
Crabapples	1 cup, 110g	84	21.9	0	0.4	0.3
Cranberries	1 cup, 110g	51	13.2	4	0.5	0.1
Cranberry Juice	½ cup, 127g	58	15.5	0.1	0.5	0.2
Currants Red And White	1 cup, 112g	63	15.5	4.8	1.6	0.2
Dates (Deglet Noor)	¼ cup, 37g	104	27.8	3	0.9	0.1
Dates Medjool Large	1 date, 24g	66	18	1.6	0.4	0
Durian	¼ cup, 61g	90	16.5	2.3	0.9	3.3
Elderberries	1 cup, 145g	106	26.7	10.2	1	0.7

FOOD	SERVING SIZE	CALORIES	TOTAL CARB (g)	FIBER (g)	PROTEIN (g)	FAT (g)
Feijoa	⅓ cup, 81g	49	12.3	5.2	0.6	0.3
Figs	1 large , 64g	47	12.3	1.9	0.5	0.2
Figs Dried	¼ cup, 37g	92	23.6	3.6	1.2	0.3
Goji Berries Dried	¼ cup, 28g	98	21.6	3.6	4	0.1
Gooseberries	1 cup, 150g	66	15.3	6.5	1.3	0.9
Gooseberries Light Syrup Pack	⅓ cup, 252g	184	47.3	6	1.6	0.5
Grape Juice	½ cup, 127g	76	18.8	0.3	0.5	0.2
Grapefruit	1 cup, 230g	74	18.6	2.5	1.4	0.2
Grapefruit California	1 cup, 230g	85	22.3	0	1.2	0.2
Grapefruit Florida	1 cup, 230g	69	17.3	2.5	1.3	0.2
Grapefruit Juice	½ cup, 120g	47	9.3	0.4	0.6	0.8
Grapefruit Pink	1 cup, 230g	97	24.5	3.7	1.8	0.3
Grapefruit Sections Water-Packed	1 cup, 244g	88	22.3	1	1.4	0.2
Grapes	1 cup, 92g	62	15.8	0.8	0.6	0.3
Grapes Muscadine	9 grape, 60g	34	8.4	2.3	0.5	0.3
Grapes Red Or Green	1 cup, 151g	104	27.3	1.4	1.1	0.2

FOOD	SERVING SIZE	CALORIES	TOTAL CARB (g)	FIBER (g)	PROTEIN (g)	FAT (g)
Groundcherries	1 cup, 140g	74	15.7	0	2.7	1
Guanabana Nectar Canned	⅓ cup, 84g	50	12.5	0.1	0.1	0.1
Guava Nectar Canned	⅓ cup, 84g	53	13.7	0.8	0.1	0.1
Guavas	1 cup, 165g	112	23.6	8.9	4.2	1.6
Jackfruit	½ cup, 83g	79	19.3	1.2	1.4	0.5
Jujube	⅓ cup, 100g	79	20.2	0	1.2	0.2
Jujube Dried	¼ cup, 35g	98	25.4	2.1	1.7	0.2
Kiwano	1 cup, 233g	103	17.6	0	4.1	2.9
Kiwifruit	1 cup, 180g	110	26.4	5.4	2.1	0.9
Kumquats	1 fruit, 19g	13	3	1.2	0.4	0.2
Lemon Juice Raw	½ cup, 122g	27	8.4	0.4	0.4	0.3
Lemons	1 cup, 212g	61	19.8	5.9	2.3	0.6
Lime Juice	½ cup, 121g	30	10.2	0.5	0.5	0.1
Limes	1 item, 67g	20	7.1	1.9	0.5	0.1
Litchis	1 cup, 190g	125	31.4	2.5	1.6	0.8
Litchis Dried	8 fruits, 20g	55	14.1	0.9	0.8	0.2

FOOD	SERVING SIZE	CALORIES	TOTAL CARB (g)	FIBER (g)	PROTEIN (g)	FAT (g)
Loganberries	1 cup, 147g	81	19.1	7.8	2.2	0.5
Longans	1 cup, 3.2g	2	0.5	0	0	0
Longans Dried	7 fruits, 12g	34	8.9	0	0.6	0
Loquats	1 cup, 149g	70	18.1	2.5	0.6	0.3
Mamey Sapote	¼ cup, 44g	55	14.1	2.4	0.6	0.2
Mango Nectar Canned	½ cup, 126g	64	16.5	0.4	0.1	0.1
Mango Pickled	1 slice, 28g	37	9.2	0.3	0.2	0.1
Mangos	½ cup, 83g	50	12.4	1.3	0.7	0.3
Mangosteen Light Syrup Pack	⅓ cup, 65g	47	11.6	1.2	0.3	0.4
Melon Cantaloupe	1 cup, 177g	60	14.4	1.6	1.5	0.3
Melon Casaba	1 cup, 170g	48	11.2	1.5	1.9	0.2
Melon Honeydew	1 cup, 170g	61	15.5	1.4	0.9	0.2
Mulberries	1 cup, 140g	60	13.7	2.4	2	0.5
Nance	1 cup, 112g	82	19	8.4	0.7	1.3
Nectarine Cooked	¼ cup, 65g	55	13.8	1	0.7	0.2
Nectarines	1 cup, 143g	63	15.1	2.4	1.5	0.5

FOOD	SERVING SIZE	CALORIES	TOTAL CARB (g)	FIBER (g)	PROTEIN (g)	FAT (g)
Oheloberries	1 cup, 140g	39	9.6	0	0.5	0.3
Olives Black	1 slice, 1g	1	0.1	0	0	0.1
Olives Green	10 olive, 27g	39	1	0.9	0.3	4.1
Olives Jumbo	1 jumbo, 15g	12	0.8	0.4	0.1	1
Orange Juice 100% Fresh	½ cup, 124g	60	14.2	0.4	0.8	0.1
Oranges	½ cup, 90g	42	10.6	2.2	0.8	0.1
Oranges California Valencia	½ cup, 90g	44	10.7	2.3	0.9	0.3
Oranges Florida	½ cup, 93g	43	10.7	2.2	0.7	0.2
Oranges Mandarin (Tangerines) Light Syrup Pack	⅓ cup, 84g	51	13.6	0.6	0.4	0.1
Oranges Navel	½ cup, 83g	41	10.4	1.8	0.8	0.1
Oranges Raw with Peel	½ cup, 85g	54	13.2	3.8	1.1	0.3
Papaya	1 cup, 145g	62	15.7	2.5	0.7	0.4
Papaya Dried	1 strip, 23g	68	17.4	1.3	0.4	0.2
Papaya Nectar Canned	⅓ cup, 84g	48	12.2	0.5	0.1	0.1
Passion Fruit	⅓ cup, 79g	77	18.5	8.2	1.7	0.6
Passion Fruit Yellow Juice	½ cup, 124g	74	17.9	0.2	0.8	0.2

FOOD	SERVING SIZE	CALORIES	TOTAL CARB (g)	FIBER (g)	PROTEIN (g)	FAT (g)
Peach Nectar	½ cup, 125g	61	14.5	0.1	0.1	0.7
Peach Pickled	½ fruit, 44g	52	12.8	0.4	0.3	0.1
Peaches Dried	¼ cup, 40g	96	24.5	3.3	1.4	0.3
Peaches Extra Light Syrup Pack	½ cup, 123g	52	13.7	1.2	0.5	0.1
Peaches Water-Packed	1 cup, 244g	59	14.9	3.2	1.1	0.1
Peaches Yellow	1 cup, 154g	60	14.7	2.3	1.4	0.4
Pear Bosc	½ cup, 70g	47	11.3	2.2	0.3	0.1
Pear Green Anjou	½ cup, 70g	46	11.1	2.2	0.3	0.1
Pear Nectar Canned	¼ cup, 63g	38	9.9	0.4	0.1	0
Pears	½ cup, 70g	40	10.7	2.2	0.3	0.1
Pears Bartlett	½ cup, 70g	44	10.5	2.2	0.3	0.1
Pears Red Anjou	1 small, 126g	78	18.8	3.8	0.4	0.2
Pears Water-Packed	½ cup, 122g	35	9.5	2	0.2	0
Persimmon Fuyu	½ fruit, 84g	59	15.6	3	0.5	0.2
Persimmons Japanese Dried	½ fruit, 17g	47	12.5	2.5	0.2	0.1
Persimmons Native Raw	1 small, 25g	32	8.4	0	0.2	0.1

FOOD	SERVING SIZE	CALORIES	TOTAL CARB (g)	FIBER (g)	PROTEIN (g)	FAT (g)
Pineapple	½ cup, 83g	42	10.9	1.2	0.4	0.1
Pineapple Canned Juice Pack Drained	½ cup, 96g	58	14.9	1.2	0.5	0.1
Pineapple Dried	¾ piece, 21g	56	14.7	0.8	0.3	0.1
Pineapple Light Syrup Pack	⅓ cup, 84g	44	11.3	0.7	0.3	0.1
Pineapple Water-Packed	½ cup, 123g	39	10.2	1	0.5	0.1
Pitanga	1 cup, 173g	57	13	0	1.4	0.7
Plantains	¼ cup, 32g	39	10.2	0.5	0.4	0.1
Plantains Cooked	¼ cup, 50g	78	20.7	1.1	0.8	0.1
Plum Java	1 cup, 135g	81	21	0	1	0.3
Plum Pickled	1 plum, 28g	34	8.6	0.3	0.1	0.1
Plums	½ cup, 83g	38	9.5	1.2	0.6	0.2
Plums Purple Water-Packed	½ cup, 124g	51	13.7	1.1	0.5	0
Pomegranate Juice Bottled	½ cup, 125g	68	16.4	0.1	0.2	0.4
Pomegranates	½ cup, 87g	72	16.3	3.5	1.5	1
Prickly Pears	1 cup, 149g	61	14.3	5.4	1.1	0.8
Prunes (Dried Plums)	3 items, 30g	72	19.2	2.1	0.7	0.1

FOOD	SERVING SIZE	CALORIES	TOTAL CARB (g)	FIBER (g)	PROTEIN (g)	FAT (g)
Pummelo	¾ cup, 142g	54	13.7	1.4	1.1	0.1
Purple Passion Fruit Juice	⅓ cup, 83g	42	11.3	0.2	0.3	0
Quinces	1 fruit, 92g	52	14.1	1.7	0.4	0.1
Raisins	1 tbsp, 10g	30	7.9	0.5	0.3	0
Raisins Golden Seedless	1 tbsp, 10g	30	8	0.3	0.3	0
Raspberries	1 cup, 123g	64	14.7	8	1.5	0.8
Raspberries Water-Packed	1 cup, 243g	85	19.4	10.7	1.9	1.1
Rhubarb	1 cup, 122g	26	5.5	2.2	1.1	0.2
Roselle	1 cup, 57g	28	6.4	0	0.5	0.4
Starfruit (Carambola)	1 cup, 132g	41	8.9	3.7	1.4	0.4
Strawberries	1 cup, 152g	49	11.7	3	1	0.5
Strawberries Water-Packed	1 cup, 242g	51	12.5	3.1	1.1	0.5
Sugar-Apples (Annona)	¼ cup, 62g	58	14.7	2.7	1.3	0.2
Tamarind Nectar Canned	1 cup, 251g	143	37	1.3	0.2	0.3
Tamarinds	¼ cup, 30g	72	18.8	1.5	0.8	0.2
Tangerine Juice	½ cup, 124g	53	12.5	0.2	0.6	0.2

FOOD	SERVING SIZE	CALORIES	TOTAL CARB (g)	FIBER (g)	PROTEIN (g)	FAT (g)
Tangerines	1 cup, 195g	103	26	3.5	1.6	0.6
Watermelon	1 cup, 154g	46	11.6	0.6	0.9	0.2
White Grapefruit	½ cup, 115g	38	9.7	1.3	0.8	0.1
Wild Blueberries	½ cup, 70g	40	9.7	3.1	0	0.1
Zante Currants	1 tbsp, 10g	29	7.7	0.4	0.3	0

7
GRAINS & CEREALS

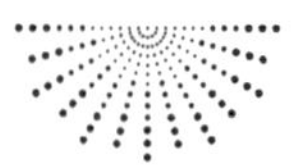

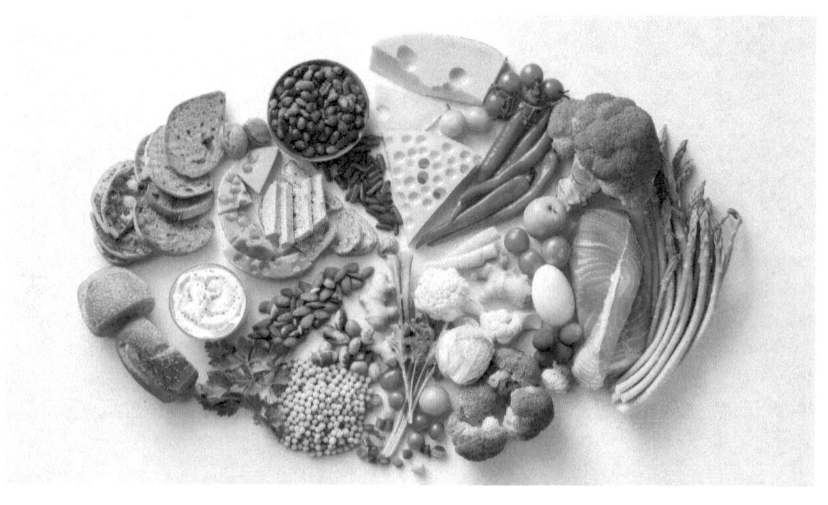

FOOD	SERVING SIZE	CALORIES	TOTAL CARB (g)	FIBER (g)	PROTEIN (g)	FAT (g)
Amaranth Cooked	½ cup, 123g	125	23	2.6	4.7	1.9
Amaranth Grain Uncooked	1 unit, 100g	371	65.3	6.7	13.6	7
Barley Cooked	½ cup, 85g	104	23.9	3.2	1.9	0.4
Barley Pearled Cooked	½ cup, 79g	97	22.3	3	1.8	0.3
Buckwheat Groats Cooked	½ cup, 85g	78	16.9	2.3	2.9	0.5
Buckwheat Groats Roasted	½ cup, 84g	77	16.7	2.3	2.8	0.5
Bulgur Cooked	½ cup, 91g	76	16.9	4.1	2.8	0.2
Corn Flour Masa	1 unit, 100g	363	76.6	6.4	8.5	3.7
Corn Flour Whole-Grain	1 unit, 100g	361	76.9	7.3	6.9	3.9
Corn Grain	1 unit, 100g	365	74.3	0	9.4	4.7
Couscous Dry	1 unit, 100g	376	77.4	5	12.8	0.6
Couscous Plain Cooked	½ cup, 80g	89	18.5	1.1	3	0.1
Gluten-Free Noodles Corn Cooked	½ cup, 70g	88	19.5	3.4	1.8	0.5

FOOD	SERVING SIZE	CALORIES	TOTAL CARB (g)	FIBER (g)	PROTEIN (g)	FAT (g)
Gluten-Free Pasta Brown Rice Flour Cooked	½ cup, 85g	117	27.4	1.4	2.9	1.4
Gluten-Free Pasta Corn and Quinoa Flour Cooked	½ cup, 83g	126	25.8	2.7	2.7	1.7
Gluten-Free Pasta Rice and Rice Bran Cooked	½ cup, 61g	122	24.9	1.2	2.6	1
Japanese Somen Cooked	½ cup, 86g	113	23.7	0	3.4	0.2
Kamut Cooked	½ cup, 86g	114	23.7	3.7	4.9	0.7
Macaroni Vegetable Cooked	½ cup, 67g	86	17.8	2.9	3	0.1
Macaroni Vegetable Dry	1 unit, 100g	367	74.9	4.3	13.1	1
Millet Cooked	½ cup, 85g	100	20	1.1	3	0.9
Millet Flour	1 unit, 100g	382	75.1	3.5	10.8	4.3
Noodles Cooked	½ cup, 80g	110	20	1	3.6	1.6
Noodles Japanese Somen Dry	1 unit, 100g	356	74.1	4.3	11.4	0.8
Noodles Rice Cooked	½ cup, 88g	95	21.1	0.9	1.6	0.2
Noodles Whole Grain Cooked	½ cup, 80g	118	23.9	3.1	4.8	1.4
Oat Bran Cooked	½ cup, 110g	44	12.6	2.9	3.5	0.9

FOOD	SERVING SIZE	CALORIES	TOTAL CARB (g)	FIBER (g)	PROTEIN (g)	FAT (g)
Oatmeal Cooked	½ cup, 117g	83	14	2	3	1.8
Pasta Cooked	½ cup, 70g	110	21.5	1.3	4	0.6
Pasta Cooked	½ cup, 62g	98	19.1	1.1	3.6	0.6
Pasta Enriched Dry	1 unit, 100g	371	74.7	3.2	13	1.5
Pasta Homemade Cooked	½ cup, 29g	38	6.8	0	1.5	0.5
Pasta Plain Fresh-Refrigerated Cooked	½ cup, 64g	84	16	0	3.3	0.7
Pasta Vegetable Cooked	½ cup, 70g	90	18.6	3	3.2	0.1
Pasta Whole Grain Cooked	½ cup, 70g	104	20.9	2.7	4.2	1.2
Quinoa Cooked	½ cup, 93g	112	19.8	2.6	4.1	1.8
Quinoa Fat Not Added in Cooking	½ cup, 85g	102	18	2.4	3.7	1.6
Quinoa Uncooked	1 unit, 100g	368	64.2	7	14.1	6.1
Rice Brown and Wild Cooked	½ cup, 76g	91	18.9	1.2	2.2	0.7
Rice Brown Cooked	½ cup, 98g	120	24.9	1.6	2.7	0.9
Rice Brown Long-Grain Raw	1 unit, 100g	367	76.3	3.6	7.5	3.2

FOOD	SERVING SIZE	CALORIES	TOTAL CARB (g)	FIBER (g)	PROTEIN (g)	FAT (g)
Rice Brown Medium-Grain Raw	1 unit, 100g	362	76.2	3.4	7.5	2.7
Rice Brown Parboiled Cooked Uncle Bens	½ cup, 78g	115	24.4	1.3	2.4	0.7
Rice White Long/Medium/Short-Grain Cooked	½ cup, 93g	121	26.6	0	2.2	0.2
Rice Wild Cooked	½ cup, 82g	83	17.5	1.5	3.3	0.3
Sorghum Grain	1 unit, 100g	329	72.1	6.7	10.6	3.5
Spaghetti Protein-Enriched Cooked	½ cup, 70g	115	21.6	1.4	6.2	0.1
Spaghetti Protein-Enriched Dry	1 unit, 100g	374	65.7	2.4	21.8	2.2
Spelt Cooked	½ cup, 97g	123	25.6	3.8	5.3	0.8
Teff Cooked	½ cup, 126g	127	25	3.5	4.9	0.8
Triticale	1 unit, 100g	336	72.1	0	13.1	2.1
Whole-Grain Cornmeal Uncooked	1 unit, 100g	362	76.9	7.3	8.1	3.6
Yellow Cornmeal Uncooked	1 unit, 100g	362	76.9	7.3	8.1	3.6
Vermicelli Made from Soybeans	½ cup, 70g	88	22	1.1	0	0

FOOD	SERVING SIZE	CALORIES	TOTAL CARB (g)	FIBER (g)	PROTEIN (g)	FAT (g)
Wheat Sprouted	1 unit, 100g	198	42.5	1.1	7.5	1.3
Whole Grain Sorghum Flour	1 unit, 100g	359	76.6	6.6	8.4	3.3
Whole Wheat Pasta	½ cup, 59g	88	17.7	2.3	3.5	1
Wild Rice Raw	1 unit, 100g	357	74.9	6.2	14.7	1.1
Yellow Cornmeal (Grits)	½ cup, 117g	76	16.2	0.8	1.4	0.5
Yellow Rice Cooked Fat Not Added	½ cup, 79g	70	15.1	0.4	1.4	0.4

8
NUTS & SEEDS

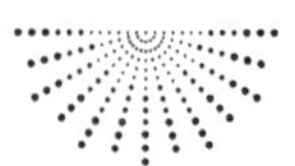

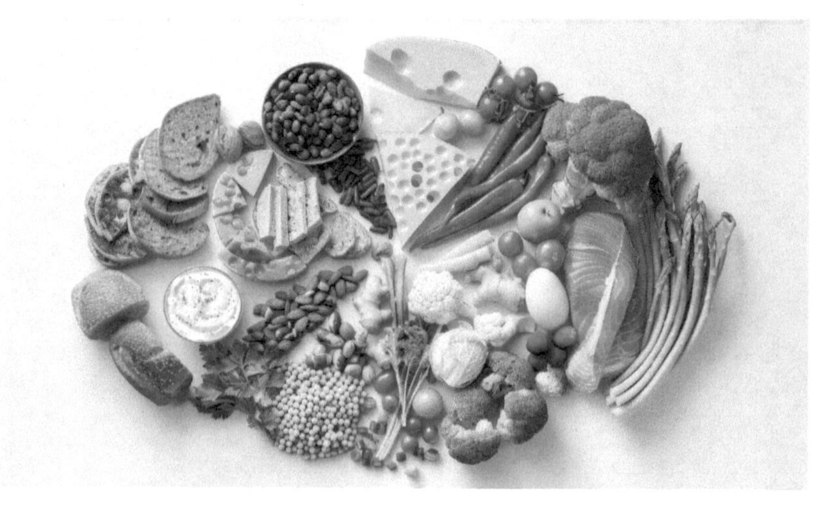

FOOD	SERVING SIZE	CALORIES	TOTAL CARB (g)	FIBER (g)	PROTEIN (g)	FAT (g)
Almond Butter	1 tbsp, 16g	98	3	1.6	3.4	8.9
Almonds "Raw, Dry Roasted, Unsalted"	1 oz, 28.4g	164	6.1	3.6	6	14.2
Black Walnuts Dried	1 oz, 28.4g	176	2.7	1.9	6.8	16.8
Brazilnuts "Raw, Dry Roasted, Unsalted"	1 oz, 28.4g	187	3.3	2.1	4.1	19.1
Butternuts Dried	1 oz, 28.4g	174	3.4	1.3	7.1	16.2
Cashew Butter	1 tbsp, 16g	94	4.4	0.3	2.8	7.9
Cashews "Raw, Dry Roasted, Unsalted"	1 oz, 28.4g	157	8.6	0.9	5.2	12.5
Chia Seeds "Raw, Dry Roasted, Unsalted"	1 oz, 28.4g	138	12	9.8	4.7	8.7
Cottonseed Kernels Roasted	1 oz, 28.4g	144	6.2	1.6	9.3	10.3
Flax Seeds "Raw, Dry Roasted, Unsalted"	1 tbsp, 10.3g	55	3	2.8	1.9	4.3
Hazelnuts "Raw, Dry Roasted, Unsalted"	1 oz, 28.4g	178	4.7	2.8	4.2	17.3
Hemp Seeds "Raw, Dry Roasted, Unsalted"	3 tbsp, 30g	166	2.6	1.2	9.5	14.6
Hickorynuts Dried	1 oz, 28.4g	187	5.2	1.8	3.6	18.3

FOOD	SERVING SIZE	CALORIES	TOTAL CARB (g)	FIBER (g)	PROTEIN (g)	FAT (g)
Mixed Nuts "Raw, Dry Roasted, Unsalted"	1 oz, 28.4g	172	6.6	2.2	4.8	15.4
Peanuts "Raw, Dry Roasted, Unsalted"	1 oz, 28.4g	167	6	2.4	6.9	14.1
Pecans "Raw, Dry Roasted, Unsalted"	1 oz, 28.4g	196	3.9	2.7	2.6	20.4
Pilinuts Dried	1 oz, 28.4g	204	1.1	0	3.1	22.6
Pine Nuts Dried	1 oz, 28.4g	179	5.5	3	3.3	17.3
Pistachio Nuts "Raw, Dry Roasted, Unsalted"	1 oz, 28.4g	159	7.7	3	5.7	12.9
Pumpkin/Squash Seeds Dried	1 oz, 28.4g	159	3	1.7	8.6	13.9
Safflower Seed Meal Partially Defatted	1 oz, 28.4g	97	13.8	0	10.1	0.7
Safflower Seeds	1 oz, 28.4g	147	9.7	0	4.6	10.9
Sesame Butter "Tahini"	1 tbsp, 15g	89	3.2	1.4	2.6	8.1
Sesame Butter Paste	1 tbsp, 16g	94	3.8	0.9	2.9	8.1
Sesame Seeds Toasted	1 oz, 28.4g	160	7.3	4	4.8	13.6
Sesame Seeds Whole Dried	1 oz, 28.4g	163	6.7	3.4	5	14.1
Sisymbrium Seeds Whole Dried	1 oz, 28.4g	90	16.5	0	3.4	1.3

FOOD	SERVING SIZE	CALORIES	TOTAL CARB (g)	FIBER (g)	PROTEIN (g)	FAT (g)
Sunflower Seed Butter	1 tbsp, 16g	99	3.7	0.9	2.8	8.8
Sunflower Seeds "Raw, Dry Roasted, Unsalted"	1 oz, 28.4g	165	6.8	3.2	5.5	14.1
Walnuts	1 oz, 28.4g	186	3.9	1.9	4.3	18.5
Watermelon Seed Kernels Dried	1 oz, 28.4g	158	4.3	0	8	13.5

9
SEAFOOD & SELFISH

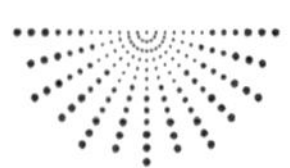

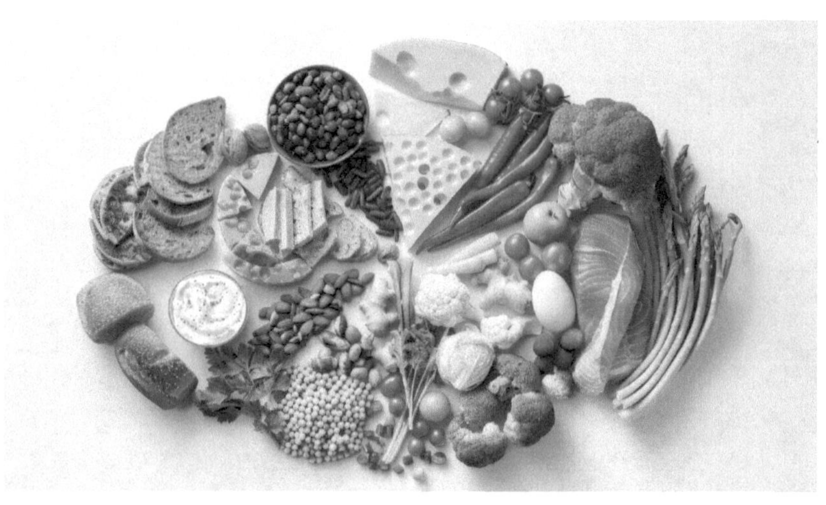

FOOD	SERVING SIZE	CALORIES	TOTAL CARB (g)	FIBER (g)	PROTEIN (g)	FAT (g)
Abalone "Steamed, baked, broiled"	4 oz, 113g	214	12.5	0	22.2	7.7
Alaska Pollock "Steamed, baked, broiled"	4 oz, 113g	125	0	0	26.5	1.3
Anchovies "Steamed, baked, broiled"	4 oz, 113g	148	0	0	23	5.5
Atlantic Cod "Steamed, baked, broiled"	4 oz, 113g	119	0	0	25.8	1
Atlantic Mackerel "Steamed, baked, broiled"	1 fillet, 113g	296	0	0	27	20.1
Atlantic Perch "Steamed, baked, broiled"	2 fillet, 113g	108	0	0	20.9	2.1
Barracuda "Steamed, baked, broiled"	1 fillet, 113g	225	0.1	0	28.6	11.2
Blue Mussels "Steamed, baked, broiled"	4 oz, 113g	194	8.4	0	26.9	5.1
Catfish "Steamed, baked, broiled"	1 fillet, 113g	170	0	0	21.6	8.4
Clams "Steamed, baked, broiled"	4 oz, 113g	167	5.8	0	28.9	2.2

FOOD	SERVING SIZE	CALORIES	TOTAL CARB (g)	FIBER (g)	PROTEIN (g)	FAT (g)
Cod "Steamed, baked, broiled"	1 fillet, 113g	98	0	0	21.7	0.6
Coho Salmon Farmed "Steamed, baked, broiled"	1 fillet, 113g	201	0	0	27.5	9.3
Coho Salmon Wild "Steamed, baked, broiled"	4 oz, 113g	157	0	0	26.5	4.9
Crab "Steamed, baked, broiled"	1 cup, 113g	115	0.1	0	24.8	1
Crayfish "Steamed, baked, broiled"	4 oz, 113g	98	0	0	19.8	1.5
Croaker "Steamed, baked, broiled"	1 fillet, 113g	148	0	0	25.3	4.5
Cuttlefish "Steamed, baked, broiled"	4 oz, 113g	179	1.9	0	36.7	1.6
Flounder "Steamed, baked, broiled"	1 fillet, 113g	99	0	0	17.6	2.7
Grouper "Steamed, baked, broiled"	4 oz, 113g	133	0	0	28.1	1.5
Haddock "Steamed, baked, broiled"	1 fillet, 113g	102	0	0	22.6	0.6
Halibut "Steamed, baked, broiled"	4 oz, 113g	125	0	0	25.5	1.8

FOOD	SERVING SIZE	CALORIES	TOTAL CARB (g)	FIBER (g)	PROTEIN (g)	FAT (g)
Herring "Steamed, baked, broiled"	4 oz, 113g	225	0.1	0	25.6	12.9
King Mackerel "Steamed, baked, broiled"	4 oz, 113g	151	0	0	29.4	2.9
Lingcod "Steamed, baked, broiled"	4 oz, 113g	123	0	0	25.6	1.5
Lobster "Steamed, baked, broiled"	1 cup, 113g	101	0	0	21.5	1
Mackerel "Steamed, baked, broiled"	1 fillet, 113g	270	0.1	0	27.2	16.9
Mullet "Steamed, baked, broiled"	1 fillet, 113g	166	0	0	27.5	5.4
Northern Pike "Steamed, baked, broiled"	4 oz, 113g	128	0	0	27.9	1
Octopus "Steamed, baked, broiled"	4 oz, 113g	185	5	0	33.7	2.4
Perch Ocean "Steamed, baked, broiled"	1 fillet, 113g	112	0	0	21.8	2.2
Perch Lake "Steamed, baked, broiled"	1 fillet, 113g	129	0	0	27.5	1.3
Pike "Steamed, baked, broiled"	1 fillet, 113g	125	0	0	27.4	1

FOOD	SERVING SIZE	CALORIES	TOTAL CARB (g)	FIBER (g)	PROTEIN (g)	FAT (g)
Pollock "Steamed, baked, broiled"	4 oz, 113g	133	0	0	28.2	1.4
Pompano "Steamed, baked, broiled"	1 fillet, 113g	238	0	0	26.8	13.7
Porgy "Steamed, baked, broiled"	1 fillet, 113g	149	0	0	26.8	3.9
Rainbow Trout "Steamed, baked, broiled"	1 fillet, 113g	190	0	0	26.9	8.3
Ray "Steamed, baked, broiled"	4 oz, 113g	184	0	0	29.8	6.4
Roe "Steamed, baked, broiled"	1 oz, 113g	231	2.2	0	32.3	9.3
Sablefish "Steamed, baked, broiled"	4 oz, 113g	283	0	0	19.4	22.2
Salmon "Steamed, baked, broiled"	1 fillet, 113g	181	0	0	29.1	6.2
Salmon "Steamed, baked, broiled"	4 oz, 113g	208	0	0	30.9	8.5
Scallops "Steamed, baked, broiled"	1 cup, 113g	155	7.2	0	27.1	1.1
Sea Bass "Steamed, baked, broiled"	1 fillet, 113g	138	0	0	26.2	2.8
Shark "Steamed, baked, broiled"	1 fillet, 113g	184	0	0	29.8	6.4

FOOD	SERVING SIZE	CALORIES	TOTAL CARB (g)	FIBER (g)	PROTEIN (g)	FAT (g)
Shrimp "Steamed, baked, broiled"	4 oz, 113g	103	1.3	0	19.6	1.5
Skipjack "Steamed, baked, broiled"	4 oz, 113g	149	0	0	31.9	1.5
Smelt "Steamed, baked, broiled"	4 oz, 113g	140	0	0	25.5	3.5
Snapper "Steamed, baked, broiled"	4 oz, 113g	145	0	0	29.7	1.9
Sockeye Salmon "Steamed, baked, broiled"	4 oz, 113g	176	0	0	29.9	6.3
Spiny Lobster "Steamed, baked, broiled"	4 oz, 113g	162	3.5	0	29.8	2.2
Squid "Steamed, baked, broiled"	4 oz, 113g	207	6.9	0	35.1	3.1
Squid Pickled	4 oz, 113g	105	3.3	0	16.9	1.5
Sturgeon "Steamed, baked, broiled"	4 oz, 113g	153	0	0	23.4	5.9
Swordfish "Steamed, baked, broiled"	4 oz, 113g	194	0	0	26.5	9
Tilapia "Steamed, baked, broiled"	1 fillet, 113g	145	0	0	29.5	3

FOOD	SERVING SIZE	CALORIES	TOTAL CARB (g)	FIBER (g)	PROTEIN (g)	FAT (g)
Tilefish "Steamed, baked, broiled"	1 fillet, 113g	166	0	0	27.7	5.3
Trout "Steamed, baked, broiled"	1 fillet, 113g	200	0	0	28.3	8.8
Tuna Bluefin "Steamed, baked, broiled"	4 oz, 113g	208	0	0	33.8	7.1
Tuna Fresh "Steamed, baked, broiled"	1 fillet, 113g	155	0	0	34.7	0.7
Turbot "Steamed, baked, broiled"	4 oz, 113g	138	0	0	23.3	4.3
Walleye Pike "Steamed, baked, broiled"	1 fillet, 113g	134	0	0	27.7	1.8
Whelk "Steamed, baked, broiled"	4 oz, 113g	311	17.5	0	53.9	0.9
Whitefish "Steamed, baked, broiled"	4 oz, 113g	194	0	0	27.7	8.5
Whiting "Steamed, baked, broiled"	1 fillet, 113g	131	0	0	26.5	1.9
Wild Atlantic Salmon Cooked	4 oz, 113g	206	0	0	28.7	9.2
Wild Eastern Oysters	4 oz, 113g	115	6.2	0	12.9	3.9

FOOD	SERVING SIZE	CALORIES	TOTAL CARB (g)	FIBER (g)	PROTEIN (g)	FAT (g)
Wolf Atlantic Cooked	1 fillet, 113g	139	0	0	25.4	3.5
Yellowfin Tuna "Steamed, baked, broiled"	4 oz, 113g	147	0	0	32.9	0.7
Yellowtail "Steamed, baked, broiled"	1 fillet, 113g	211	0	0	33.5	7.6

10

VEGETABLES & VEGETABLE PRODUCTS

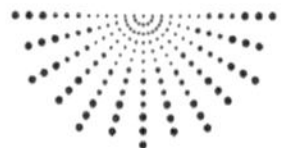

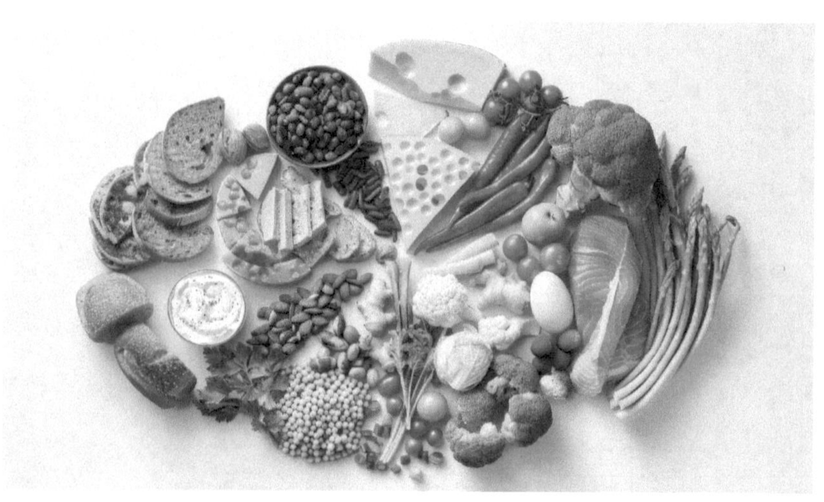

FOOD	SERVING SIZE	CALORIES	TOTAL CARB (g)	FIBER (g)	PROTEIN (g)	FAT (g)
Acorn Squash Raw	½ cup, 70 g	28	7.3	1.1	0.6	0.1
Acorn Squash, Baked	½ cup, 103 g	57.7	15	4.5	1.2	0.1
Acorn Squash, Cooked	½ cup, 122 g	41.5	10.7	3.2	0.8	0.1
Alfalfa Sprouts	1 cup, 33 g	7.6	0.7	0.6	1.3	0.2
Amaranth Leaves Raw	1 cup, 28 g	6.4	1.1	0	0.7	0.1
Arrowhead Raw	1 large, 25 g	24.8	5.1	0	1.3	0.1
Arrowroot	½ cup, 60 g	39	8	0.8	2.5	0.1
Artichokes Globe	1 item, 128 g	60.2	13.5	6.9	4.2	0.2
Artichokes Globe, Cooked	½ cup, 84 g	37.8	7.7	3.9	2.6	0.4
Arugula	10 leaf, 20 g	5	0.7	0.3	0.5	0.1
Asparagus	1 cup, 134 g	26.8	5.2	2.8	2.9	0.2
Asparagus, Cooked	½ cup, 90 g	19.8	3.7	1.8	2.2	0.2
Baby Carrots	6 large, 90 g	31.5	7.4	2.6	0.6	0.1

FOOD	SERVING SIZE	CALORIES	TOTAL CARB (g)	FIBER (g)	PROTEIN (g)	FAT (g)
Bamboo Shoots	1 cup, 151 g	40.8	7.9	3.3	3.9	0.5
Beet Greens Cooked	½ cup, 75 g	34.5	3.9	2.1	1.9	1.9
Beet Greens, Raw	1 cup, 38 g	8.4	1.6	1.4	0.8	0
Beets Cooked	½ cup, 85 g	37.4	8.4	1.7	1.4	0.2
Beets, Raw	1 cup, 136 g	58.5	13	3.8	2.2	0.2
Bell Peppers Green	1 cup, 149 g	29.8	6.9	2.5	1.3	0.3
Bell Peppers Green, Cooked	½ cup, 68 g	19	4.6	0.8	0.6	0.1
Bell Peppers Red, Cooked	½ cup, 68 g	19	4.6	0.8	0.6	0.1
Bitter Melon	1 cup, 93 g	15.8	3.4	2.6	0.9	0.2
Bitter Melon, Cooked	½ cup, 62 g	11.8	2.7	1.2	0.5	0.1
Bok Choy	1 cup, 70 g	9.1	1.5	0.7	1.1	0.1
Borage Raw	1 cup, 89 g	18.7	2.7	0	1.6	0.6
Broccoflower Cooked	1 cup, 87 g	51.3	5.2	2.7	2.5	3.1
Broccoli	1 cup, 91 g	30.9	6	2.4	2.6	0.3

FOOD	SERVING SIZE	CALORIES	TOTAL CARB (g)	FIBER (g)	PROTEIN (g)	FAT (g)
Broccoli Chinese, Cooked	1 cup, 88 g	19.4	3.4	2.2	1	0.6
Broccoli Raab Raw	1 cup, 40 g	8.8	1.1	1.1	1.3	0.2
Broccoli Raab, Cooked	1 cup, 85 g	21.3	2.7	2.4	3.3	0.4
Broccoli Stalks Raw	1 stalk, 114 g	31.9	6	0	3.4	0.4
Broccoli, Cooked	½ cup, 78 g	27.3	5.6	2.6	1.9	0.3
Brussels Sprouts, Cooked	5 item, 105 g	37.8	7.5	2.7	2.7	0.5
Brussels Sprouts, Raw	1 cup, 88 g	37.8	7.9	3.3	3	0.3
Burdock Root Raw	1 cup, 118 g	85	20.5	3.9	1.8	0.2
Burdock Root, Cooked	½ cup, 63 g	55.4	13.3	1.1	1.3	0.1
Butterbur Raw	1 cup, 94 g	13.2	3.4	0	0.4	0
Cabbage Chinese Cooked	½ cup, 88 g	30.8	1.5	0.9	1.3	2.4
Cabbage Chinese Raw	1 cup, 76 g	12.2	2.5	0.9	0.9	0.2
Cabbage Common Raw	½ cup, 35 g	8.4	1.9	0.8	0.4	0.1
Cabbage Green Cooked	½ cup, 78 g	32.8	4.1	1.4	1	1.8

FOOD	SERVING SIZE	CALORIES	TOTAL CARB (g)	FIBER (g)	PROTEIN (g)	FAT (g)
Cabbage Napa, Cooked	½ cup, 109 g	13.1	2.4	0	1.2	0.2
Cabbage Red	1 cup, 89 g	27.6	6.6	1.9	1.3	0.1
Cabbage Red Cooked	½ cup, 78 g	36.7	5.2	2	1.1	1.8
Cabbage Savoy	1 cup, 70 g	18.9	4.3	2.2	1.4	0.1
Cabbage Savoy Cooked	½ cup, 75 g	36	4.6	2.3	1.5	1.8
Cabbage Swamp, Cooked	1 cup, 98 g	19.6	3.6	1.9	2	0.2
Cactus Cooked	½ cup, 77 g	26.2	2.4	1.5	1	1.7
Calabash Raw	½ cup, 58 g	8.1	2	0.3	0.4	0
Calabaza Cooked	½ cup, 83 g	37.4	6.6	2.3	0.9	1.4
Cardoon Raw	1 cup, 178 g	30.3	7.2	2.8	1.2	0.2
Carrots	1 cup, 128 g	52.5	12.3	3.6	1.2	0.3
Carrots Cooked	6 baby, 36 g	20.2	2.7	1.2	0.2	1.1
Cassava	½ cup, 103 g	164.8	39.2	1.9	1.4	0.3
Cassava Cooked	3 item, 60 g	105.6	22.2	1.1	0.8	1.5

FOOD	SERVING SIZE	CALORIES	TOTAL CARB (g)	FIBER (g)	PROTEIN (g)	FAT (g)
Cauliflower	1 cup, 107 g	26.8	5.3	2.1	2.1	0.3
Cauliflower, Cooked	½ cup, 62 g	14.3	2.5	1.4	1.1	0.3
Celeriac	1 cup, 156 g	65.5	14.4	2.8	2.3	0.5
Celeriac Cooked	½ cup, 78 g	34.3	7.5	1.5	1.2	0.2
Celery	1 cup, 101 g	14.1	3	1.6	0.7	0.2
Celery Cooked	½ cup, 78 g	28.9	3	1.2	0.6	1.8
Celtuce	10 leaf, 80 g	14.4	2.9	1.4	0.7	0.2
Chard Cooked	½ cup, 75 g	27	3	1.5	1.4	1.5
Chayote Fruit Raw	1 cup, 132 g	25.1	6	2.2	1.1	0.2
Chestnut Water	1 cup, 158 g	123.2	30.4	6.2	2.2	0.1
Chicory Greens	1 cup, 29 g	6.7	1.4	1.2	0.5	0.1
Chicory Roots	1 root, 60 g	43.2	10.5	0.9	0.8	0.1
Chili Peppers Green	1 cup, 139 g	29.2	6.4	2.4	1	0.4
Christophine Cooked	½ cup, 83 g	34.9	4.1	2.2	0.5	2.1

FOOD	SERVING SIZE	CALORIES	TOTAL CARB (g)	FIBER (g)	PROTEIN (g)	FAT (g)
Chrysanthemum Leaves	1 cup, 51 g	12.2	1.5	1.5	1.7	0.3
Collards	1 cup, 36 g	11.5	2	1.4	1.1	0.2
Collards, Cooked	½ cup, 85 g	28.1	4.8	3.4	2.3	0.6
Corn Cooked	½ cup, 85 g	81.6	15.9	2	2.1	2.3
Corn Dried, Cooked	½ cup, 112 g	122.1	17.2	1.8	2.4	6.1
Cress Cooked	½ cup, 70 g	30.8	2.6	0.5	1.3	2.1
Crookneck Summer Squash	1 cup, 127 g	24.1	4.9	1.3	1.3	0.3
Crookneck Summer Squash, Cooked	½ cup, 90 g	17.1	3.4	1	0.9	0.4
Cucumber Cooked	½ cup, 93 g	39.1	4	0.6	0.7	2.7
Cucumber Peeled Raw	1 cup, 133 g	13.3	2.9	0.9	0.8	0.2
Dandelion Greens	1 cup, 55 g	24.8	5.1	1.9	1.5	0.4
Dandelion Greens, Cooked	½ cup, 53 g	17.5	3.4	1.5	1.1	0.3
Dasheen Boiled	½ cup, 72 g	101.5	24.8	3.7	0.4	0.1
Dill Pickles	2 small, 70 g	8.4	1.7	0.7	0.4	0.2

FOOD	SERVING SIZE	CALORIES	TOTAL CARB (g)	FIBER (g)	PROTEIN (g)	FAT (g)
Dock Raw	1 cup, 133 g	29.3	4.3	3.9	2.7	0.9
Drumstick Leaves Raw	1 cup, 21 g	13.4	1.7	0.4	2	0.3
Drumstick Pods Raw	1 cup, 100 g	37	8.5	3.2	2.1	0.2
Drumstick Pods, Cooked	½ cup, 59 g	21.2	4.8	2.5	1.2	0.1
Edamame Unprepared	1 cup, 118 g	128.6	9	5.7	13.2	5.6
Eggplant	1 cup, 82 g	20.5	4.8	2.5	0.8	0.1
Eggplant, Cooked	½ cup, 50 g	17.5	4.4	1.3	0.4	0.1
Endive	1 cup, 50 g	8.5	1.7	1.6	0.6	0.1
Eppaw Raw	1 cup, 100 g	150	31.7	0	4.6	1.8
Escarole, Cooked	½ cup, 75 g	11.3	2.3	2.1	0.9	0.1
Fennel	1 cup, 87 g	27	6.4	2.7	1.1	0.2
Fennel Bulb Cooked	½bulb, 106 g	51.9	12.2	5.2	2.1	0.3
Fireweed Leaves Raw	1 cup, 23 g	23.7	4.4	2.4	1.1	0.6
Fungi Cloud Ears, Dried	1 cup, 28 g	79.5	20.4	19.6	2.6	0.2

FOOD	SERVING SIZE	CALORIES	TOTAL CARB (g)	FIBER (g)	PROTEIN (g)	FAT (g)
Garden Cress	1 cup, 50 g	16	2.8	0.6	1.3	0.4
Garden Cress, Cooked	½ cup, 68 g	15.6	2.6	0.5	1.3	0.4
Gourd Dishcloth, Raw	1 cup, 95 g	19	4.1	1	1.1	0.2
Grape Leaves Canned	9 item, 40 g	27.6	4.7	4	1.7	0.8
Green Banana Cooked	1 small, 54 g	47.5	12.3	1.4	0.6	0.2
Green Plantains Boiled	1 slice, 27 g	31.3	8.4	0.6	0.2	0
Jerusalem-Artichokes Raw	1 cup, 150 g	109.5	26.2	2.4	3	0
Jews Ear	1 cup, 99 g	24.8	6.7	0	0.5	0
Jute Potherb Raw	1 cup, 28 g	9.5	1.6	0	1.3	0.1
Jute Potherb, Cooked	½ cup, 44 g	16.3	3.2	0.9	1.6	0.1
Kale, Cooked	½ cup, 65 g	23.4	3.4	2.6	1.9	0.8
Kohlrabi	1 cup, 135 g	36.5	8.4	4.9	2.3	0.1
Kohlrabi, Cooked	½ cup, 82 g	23.8	5.5	0.9	1.5	0.1
Lambsquarter Cooked	½ cup, 90 g	28.8	4.5	1.9	2.9	0.6

FOOD	SERVING SIZE	CALORIES	TOTAL CARB (g)	FIBER (g)	PROTEIN (g)	FAT (g)
Leaf Lettuce Green	1 cup, 36 g	5.4	1	0.5	0.5	0.1
Leeks	1 cup, 89 g	54.3	12.6	1.6	1.3	0.3
Leeks, Cooked	½ cup, 62 g	19.2	4.7	0.6	0.5	0.1
Lettuce Iceberg	1 cup, 72 g	10.1	2.1	0.9	0.6	0.1
Lettuce Red Leaf	1 cup, 28 g	3.6	0.6	0.3	0.4	0.1
Lettuce Romaine	1 cup, 47 g	8	1.5	1	0.6	0.1
Lotus Root	9 slice, 81 g	59.9	14	4	2.1	0.1
Lotus Root, Cooked	½ cup, 60 g	39.6	9.6	1.9	0.9	0
Mushrooms Shiitake, Dried	5 item, 20 g	59.2	15.1	2.3	1.9	0.2
Mushrooms Chantarelle	1 cup diced, 54 g	17.3	3.7	2.1	0.8	0.3
Mushrooms Cremini	1 cup, 87 g	19.1	3.7	0.5	2.2	0.1
Mushrooms Enoki	5 item, 25 g	9.3	2	0.7	0.7	0.1
Mushrooms Maitake	1 cup, 70 g	21.7	4.9	1.9	1.4	0.1

FOOD	SERVING SIZE	CALORIES	TOTAL CARB (g)	FIBER (g)	PROTEIN (g)	FAT (g)
Mushrooms Morel	1 cup diced, 66 g	20.5	3.4	1.8	2.1	0.4
Mushrooms Portobellos	1 cup, 86 g	18.9	3.3	1.1	1.8	0.3
Mushrooms Portobellos Grilled	1 cup, 121 g	35.1	5.4	2.7	4	0.7
Mushrooms Shiitake, Cooked	½ cup, 74 g	41.4	10.6	1.6	1.2	0.2
Mushrooms White Button, Cooked	½ cup, 78 g	21.8	4.1	1.7	1.7	0.4
Mustard Greens	1 cup, 56 g	15.1	2.6	1.8	1.6	0.2
Mustard Greens, Cooked	½ cup, 70 g	18.2	3.2	1.4	1.8	0.3
Mustard Spinach	1 cup, 150 g	33	5.9	4.2	3.3	0.5
Mustard Spinach, Cooked	½ cup, 90 g	14.4	2.5	1.8	1.5	0.2
New Zealand Spinach Cooked	½ cup, 90 g	10.8	1.9	1.3	1.2	0.2
Nopales	1 cup, 86 g	13.8	2.9	1.9	1.1	0.1
Nopales, Cooked	½ cup, 75 g	11.3	2.5	1.5	1	0
Okra	1 cup, 100 g	33	7.5	3.2	1.9	0.2

FOOD	SERVING SIZE	CALORIES	TOTAL CARB (g)	FIBER (g)	PROTEIN (g)	FAT (g)
Okra, Cooked	½ cup, 40 g	8.8	1.8	1	0.7	0.1
Onions	1 cup, 160 g	64	14.9	2.7	1.8	0.2
Onions Green Cooked	½ cup, 112 g	59.4	8.4	2.9	2.1	2.9
Onions Pearl Cooked	½ cup, 93 g	26	6.2	1.3	0.7	0
Onions, Cooked	½ cup, 105 g	46.2	10.7	1.5	1.4	0.2
Pak-Choi Cooked	½ cup, 85 g	10.2	1.5	0.9	1.3	0.1
Palm Hearts Canned	1 cup, 146 g	40.9	6.7	3.5	3.7	0.9
Parsnips	1 cup, 133 g	99.8	23.9	6.5	1.6	0.4
Parsnips, Cooked	½ cup, 78 g	55.4	13.3	2.8	1	0.2
Pepper Raw	1 item, 45 g	10.8	2.3	0.8	0.4	0.1
Pepper Sweet Red Raw	1 item, 45 g	14	2.7	0.9	0.4	0.1
Peppers Chili Red	1 item, 45 g	18	4	0.7	0.8	0.2
Peppers Green Cooked	½ cup, 71 g	34.1	4.6	0.9	0.6	1.9
Peppers Hot Green Chili	1 item, 45 g	18	4.3	0.7	0.9	0.1

FOOD	SERVING SIZE	CALORIES	TOTAL CARB (g)	FIBER (g)	PROTEIN (g)	FAT (g)
Plantain Boiled	1 slice, 27 g	31.3	8.4	0.6	0.2	0
Plantain Fried	1 slice, 27 g	65.1	11	0.8	0.4	2.7
Poke Greens Cooked	½ cup, 80 g	29.6	2.4	1.1	1.8	1.9
Poke Raw	1 cup, 160 g	36.8	5.9	2.7	4.2	0.6
Potato	1 baby, 60 g	75	12.3	0.8	1.1	2.5
Potato Baked	½ cup, 115 g	107	24.7	1.7	2.2	0.1
Potato Boiled	1 baby, 60 g	75	12.3	0.8	1.1	2.5
Potato Roasted	1 baby, 60 g	75	12.3	0.8	1.1	2.5
Potatoes Boiled	½ cup, 78 g	67.9	15.7	1.4	1.5	0.1
Potatoes Red Flesh and Skin Raw	½ cup, 75 g	52.5	11.9	1.3	1.4	0.1
Potatoes Russet Flesh and Skin Raw	½ cup, 75 g	59.3	13.6	1	1.6	0.1
Potatoes Sweet	1 cup, 133 g	114.4	26.8	4	2.1	0.1
Potatoes Sweet Mashed	½ cup, 127 g	128.3	29.5	2.2	2.5	0.3
Potatoes Sweet, Boiled	½ cup, 164 g	124.6	29.1	4.1	2.2	0.2

FOOD	SERVING SIZE	CALORIES	TOTAL CARB (g)	FIBER (g)	PROTEIN (g)	FAT (g)
Potatoes Sweet, Cooked	½ cup, 100 g	90	20.7	3.3	2	0.2
Potatoes White Flesh and Skin Raw	½ cup, 75 g	51.8	11.8	1.8	1.3	0.1
Pumpkin Raw	1 cup, 116 g	30.2	7.5	0.6	1.2	0.1
Pumpkin, Cooked	½ cup, 123 g	24.6	6	1.4	0.9	0.1
Purslane	1 cup, 43 g	8.6	1.5	0	0.9	0.2
Purslane, Cooked	½ cup, 58 g	10.4	2.1	0	0.9	0.1
Radicchio	1 cup, 40 g	9.2	1.8	0.4	0.6	0.1
Radish Daikon Cooked	½ cup, 77 g	33.1	2.5	1.2	0.5	2.5
Radish Sprouts	1 cup, 38 g	16.3	1.4	0	1.4	1
Radishes	1 cup, 116 g	18.6	3.9	1.9	0.8	0.1
Radishes Oriental	1 cup, 116 g	20.9	4.8	1.9	0.7	0.1
Radishes Oriental Dried	1 cup, 116 g	314.4	73.5	27.7	9.2	0.8
Radishes Oriental, Cooked	½ cup, 74 g	12.6	2.5	1.2	0.5	0.2
Rutabagas raw	1 cup, 140 g	51.8	12.1	3.2	1.5	0.2

FOOD	SERVING SIZE	CALORIES	TOTAL CARB (g)	FIBER (g)	PROTEIN (g)	FAT (g)
Rutabagas, Cooked	½ cup, 85 g	25.5	5.8	1.5	0.8	0.2
Salsify Cooked	½ cup, 70 g	60.9	10.3	2.1	1.8	1.8
Salsify Raw	1 cup, 133 g	109.1	24.7	4.4	4.4	0.3
Sauerkraut	1 cup, 142 g	27	6.1	4.1	1.3	0.2
Seaweed Raw	1 cup, 80 g	30.4	6.7	0.6	1.9	0.2
Spinach	1 cup, 30 g	6.9	1.1	0.7	0.9	0.1
Spinach New Zealand	1 cup, 56 g	7.8	1.4	0.8	0.8	0.1
Spinach, Cooked	½ cup, 90 g	20.7	3.4	2.2	2.7	0.2
Spirulina Seaweed, Dried	½ cup, 56 g	162.4	13.4	2	32.2	4.3
Spring Onions	1 cup, 100 g	32	7.3	2.6	1.8	0.2
Squash Butternut	1 cup, 140 g	63	16.4	2.8	1.4	0.1
Squash Butternut, Cooked	½ cup, 103 g	41.2	10.8	3.3	0.9	0.1
Squash Hubbard	1 cup, 116 g	46.4	10.1	4.5	2.3	0.6
Squash Scallop	1 cup, 130 g	23.4	5	1.6	1.6	0.3

FOOD	SERVING SIZE	CALORIES	TOTAL CARB (g)	FIBER (g)	PROTEIN (g)	FAT (g)
Squash Spaghetti	1 cup, 101 g	31.3	7	1.5	0.6	0.6
Squash Spaghetti, Cooked	½ cup, 77 g	20.8	5	1.1	0.5	0.2
Squash Summer	½ cup, 57 g	9.1	1.9	0.6	0.7	0.1
Squash Summer, Cooked	½ cup, 90 g	18	3.9	1.3	0.8	0.3
Squash Winter, Cooked	½ cup, 103 g	38.1	9.1	2.9	0.9	0.4
Squash Zucchini Baby Raw	5 small, 80 g	16.8	2.5	0.9	2.2	0.3
Swiss Chard, Cooked	½ cup, 88 g	17.6	3.6	1.8	1.7	0.1
Tannier Cooked	½ cup, 95 g	145.4	34.4	5.3	1.9	0.3
Taro	1 cup, 104 g	116.5	27.5	4.3	1.6	0.2
Taro Baked	1 cup, 132 g	190.1	45	7	2.5	0.3
Taro Leaves Raw	1 cup, 28 g	11.8	1.9	1	1.4	0.2
Taro Shoots Raw	½ cup, 43 g	4.7	1	0	0.4	0
Taro Tahitian, Cooked	½ cup, 69 g	30.4	4.7	0	2.9	0.5
Taro, Cooked	½ cup, 66 g	93.7	22.8	3.4	0.3	0.1

FOOD	SERVING SIZE	CALORIES	TOTAL CARB (g)	FIBER (g)	PROTEIN (g)	FAT (g)
Tomatoes Raw	1 cup, 149 g	26.8	5.8	1.8	1.3	0.3
Tomatoes, Cooked	½ cup, 120 g	21.6	4.8	0.8	1.1	0.1
Turnip Greens	1 cup, 55 g	17.6	3.9	1.8	0.8	0.2
Turnip Greens, Cooked	½ cup, 72 g	14.4	3.1	2.5	0.8	0.2
Turnips	1 cup, 130 g	36.4	8.4	2.3	1.2	0.1
Turnips, Cooked	½ cup, 78 g	17.2	3.9	1.6	0.6	0.1
Wasabi Root	½ cup, 65 g	70.9	15.3	5.1	3.1	0.4
Waterchestnuts Chinese Raw	½ cup, 62 g	60.1	14.8	1.9	0.9	0.1
Watercress	1 cup, 34 g	3.7	0.4	0.2	0.8	0
Watercress Cooked	½ cup, 69 g	7.6	0.9	0.3	1.6	0.1
Yam	1 cup, 150 g	177	41.8	6.2	2.3	0.3
Yam, Cooked	½ cup, 68 g	78.9	18.7	2.7	1	0.1
Zucchini	1 cup, 124 g	21.1	3.9	1.2	1.5	0.4
Zucchini, Cooked	½ cup, 90 g	13.5	2.4	0.9	1	0.3

THE GI, GL & NET CARB COUNTER

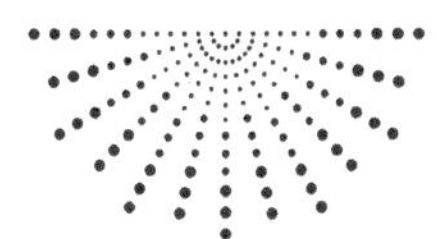

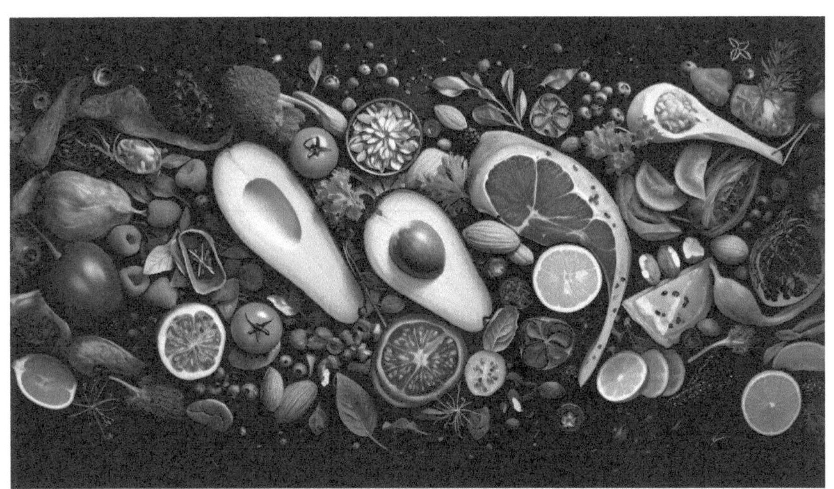

1

INTRODUCTION TO THE GLYCEMIC INDEX AND GLYCEMIC LOAD COUNTER

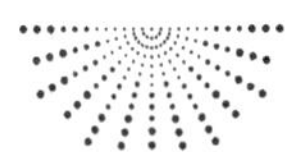

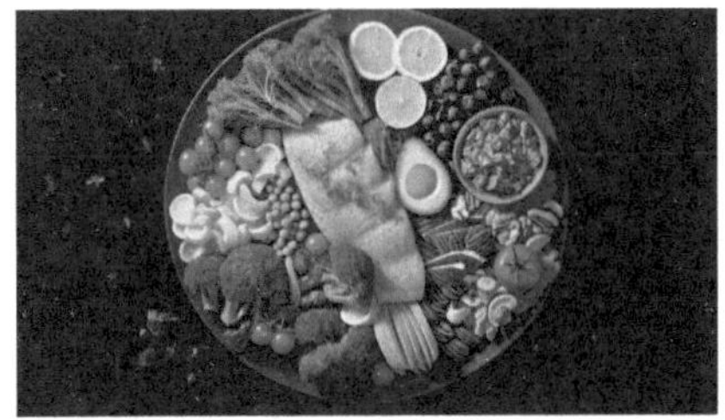

INTRODUCTION TO THE GI, GL & NET CARB COUNTER

The GI, GL & Net Carb counter is a pivotal tool in implementing tier 3 of the Low GL Diabetes Diet, designed to maximize the health benefits of this effective approach. Unlike other counters that may include foods unsuitable for diabetes or overall health—such as highly processed foods, foods high in advanced glycation end-products (AGEs), sodium, or cholesterol—this counter focuses exclusively on what truly matters for health management. It emphasizes initially healthy-looking foods, necessitating further investigation to determine their suitability for the diet.

Through rigorous evaluation, we have refined an initial list of over 4,000 foods, applying strict criteria aligned with the principles of a Low Glycemic Load (GL) Diabetes Diet. Our selection process involved excluding foods inherently unsuitable for a diabetes-friendly diet—those high in processed content, added sugars, sodium, and unhealthy fats, and those prepared through methods not compliant with dietary recommendations, such as frying and breading. This meticulous process has significantly narrowed the list to 1,100, removing over 2,900+ irrelevant or potentially harmful choices for managing diabetes.

This leads us to question: Are all foods listed here unequivocally diabetes-friendly? The answer depends on their Glycemic Load (GL). Our primary objective extends beyond merely cataloging diabetes-friendly foods; it aims to provide comprehensive information about each "potentially diabetes-friendly" food's Glycemic Index (GI), Glycemic Load (GL), net carbohydrate content and recommended serving sizes. The term "potentially" is crucial, indicating that the GI and GL metrics provide a nuanced understanding that moves beyond generic labels like "whole food" or "minimally processed food."

For example, the section "Beef, Veal, Pork, Lamb & Fish" was removed due to its minimal relevance to carbohydrate content. Instead, the volume "The Diabetes-Friendly Carbs, Proteins, Fats, and Fiber Counter" has two dedicated chapters—one for meat and another for seafood and shellfish.

This precise and in-depth approach ensures you are equipped to make informed food choices. Our counter, tailored specifically for the Low GL Diabetes Diet, highlights only those foods that seem potentially beneficial for individuals managing diabetes and that require validation through the GI & GL Framework. For instance, items like Tapioca Pearl (Dry), Wheat Durum, Egg Noodles, and Semolina have been excluded due to processing that alters their nutritional value. This discerning process has eliminated many unhealthy options, making our counter more relevant, precise, and user-friendly.

COUNTER STRUCTURE

The counter is organized into 12 primary food categories to simplify navigation and selection:

- Breads and Baked Products
- Beans & Lentils
- Beverages
- Dairy products
- Dairy Alternatives — Plant-based Options
- Dressings & Oils
- Fruits
- Fruit Products
- Grains, Cereals, Pasta & Rice
- Herbs and Spices
- Nuts & seeds
- Vegetables & Vegetable Products

This structure lets users quickly locate and choose from various healthy options within each essential food group.

USING THE COUNTER

1. **Select From Food Groups:** Begin with any MyPlate.gov food groups: fruits, vegetables, grains, proteins, and dairy. Items within the 12 categories are alphabetically listed for easy reference.
2. **Prioritize Glycemic Load (GL):** Focus on foods classified as having a low Glycemic Load (GL) for your daily diet. Foods with a medium GL, ranging between 10 and 19, can

occasionally be included to diversify your dietary choices without significantly impacting your blood sugar levels.

3. **Adapt the Serving Sizes - Maintain Carbohydrate Intake:** It's crucial to adapt the counter's specified serving sizes to keep net carbohydrates under 15 grams per serving. This practice is essential for managing carbohydrate intake and eating appropriately for your dietary goals.
4. **Choose Low GL Options:** When selecting within a food subcategory and considering your preferences, opt for the item with the lowest GL. Understanding the direct physiological impact of GL values is essential: 1 GL unit is equivalent to the effect of consuming 1 gram of pure glucose. Thus, choosing the lowest GL option within your preferences is crucial for maintaining stable blood sugar levels.
5. **Balance Your Diet:** In addition to focusing on GL and net carbs, maintaining a balanced diet is crucial. Incorporate a variety of foods from all categories to fulfill overall nutritional requirements, reinforcing the dietary guidelines and meal planning principles introduced earlier.

By presenting a streamlined selection, we aim to simplify dietary decision-making and aid in managing diabetes efficiently and confidently.

2

BREADS AND BAKED PRODUCTS

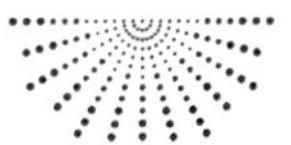

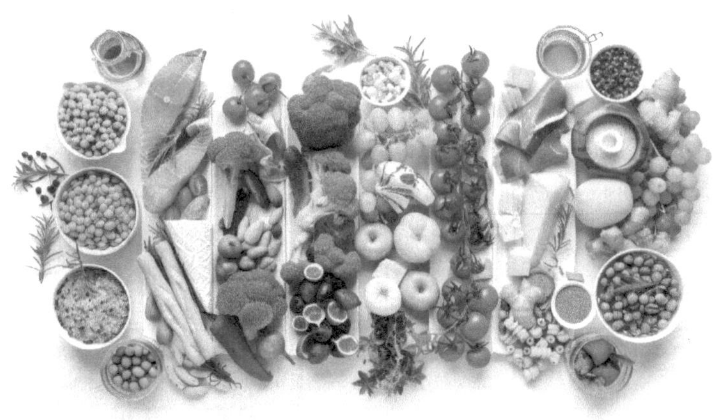

BAKED FOODS & BREADS	SERVING SIZE	NET CARB (g)	GI VALUE	GI LEVEL	GL VALUE	GL LEVEL
Almond Flour Bread	1 slice, 25g	3	35	Low	1.1	Low
Apple Pie	1 slice, 125g	32	70	High	22.4	High
Apple Turnover	1 med., 100g	33	45	Low	14.9	Med.
Baguette	1 serv., 50g	25	95	High	23.8	High
Bakewell Tart	1 slice, 80g	35	76	High	26.6	High
Baklava	1 piece, 33g	29	85	High	24.7	High
Barley Bread	1 slice, 25g	12	34	Low	4.1	Med.
Beignets	1 med., 60g	34	81	High	27.5	High
Biscotti	1 biscotti, 20g	12	70	High	8.4	Low
Biscuit Sandwiches	1 sandwich, 130g	28	70	High	19.6	High
Black Forest Cake	1 slice, 100g	34	74	High	25.2	High
Black Forest Tart	1 slice, 100g	25	76	High	19	Med.
Blackberry Pie	1 slice, 125g	29	70	High	20.3	High
Blueberry Custard Tart	1 slice, 100g	21	76	High	16	Med.

BAKED FOODS & BREADS	SERVING SIZE	NET CARB (g)	GI VALUE	GI LEVEL	GL VALUE	GL LEVEL
Boston Cream Pie	1 slice, 100g	34	70	High	23.8	High
Brioche	1 slice, 30g	15	82	High	12.3	Med.
Buckwheat Bread	1 slice, 25g	15	47	Low	7.1	Low
Butter Cookies	1 cookie, 30g	11	73	High	8	Low
Buttermilk Biscuits	1 biscuit, 64g	24	70	High	16.8	Med.
Buttermilk Pie	1 slice, 125g	38	70	High	26.6	High
Cannoli	1 med., 85g	32	75	High	24	High
Carrot Cake	1 slice, 100g	40	74	High	29.6	High
Cheesecake	1 slice, 100g	28	74	High	20.7	High
Cherry Pie	1 slice, 125g	31	70	High	21.7	High
Chocolate Cake	1 slice, 100g	35	74	High	25.9	High
Chocolate Chip Biscuits	1 biscuit, 57g	33	70	High	23.1	High
Chocolate Chip Cookies	1 cookie, 30g	19	73	High	13.9	Med.
Chocolate Pecan Pie	1 slice, 125g	42	70	High	29.4	High

BAKED FOODS & BREADS	SERVING SIZE	NET CARB (g)	GI VALUE	GI LEVEL	GL VALUE	GL LEVEL
Chocolate Tart	1 slice, 100g	23	76	High	17.5	Med.
Churros	1 med., 30g	24	82	High	19.7	High
Ciabatta	1 serv., 50g	20	78	High	15.6	Med.
Cinnamon Roll	1 small, 60g	31	82	High	25.4	High
Cinnamon Roll Biscuits	1 biscuit, 28g	20	70	High	14	Med.
Coconut Cake	1 slice, 80g	31	74	High	22.9	High
Coconut Cream Pie	1 slice, 100g	26	70	High	18.2	Med.
Coconut Flour Bread	1 slice, 25g	2	45	Low	0.9	Low
Coffee Cake	1 slice, 100g	38	74	High	28.1	High
Corn Tortilla	1 med., 55g	13	70	High	9.1	Low
Cornbread	1 piece, 60g	28	65	Med.	18.2	Med.
Cornish Pasty	1 small, 150g	40	83	High	33.2	High
Croissant	1 med.,57g	23	81	High	18.6	Med.
Custard Tart	1 slice, 100g	20	76	High	15.2	Med.
Danish Pastry	1 med., 84g	37	85	High	31.5	High

BAKED FOODS & BREADS	SERVING SIZE	NET CARB (g)	GI VALUE	GI LEVEL	GL VALUE	GL LEVEL
Dobos Torte	1 slice, 100g	31	81	High	25.1	High
Double Chocolate Cookies	1 cookie, 30g	19	73	High	13.9	Med.
Drop Biscuits	1 biscuit, 30g	11	70	High	7.7	Low
Eccles Cake	1 Cake, 60g	27	74	High	20	High
Éclair	1 med., 85g	26	88	High	22.9	High
Empanada	1 small, 100g	35	75	High	26.3	High
Ezekiel Bread	1 slice, 25g	12	36	Low	4.3	Low
Flaxseed Bread	1 slice, 25g	10	45	Low	4.5	Low
Focaccia	1 slice, 50g	20	72	High	14.4	Med.
Fougasse	1 serv., 50g	20	71	High	14.2	Med.
French Bread	1 slice, 30g	15	95	High	14.3	Med.
Garlic Butter Biscuits	1 biscuit, 25g	10	70	High	7	Low
German Chocolate Cake	1 slice, 100g	38	74	High	28.1	High
Gingerbread Cookies	1 cookie, 30g	16	73	High	11.7	Med.
Gluten-Free Multiseed Bread	1 slice, 25g	11	55	Low	6.1	Low
Green Onion Biscuits	1 biscuit, 28g	14	70	High	9.8	Low

BAKED FOODS & BREADS	SERVING SIZE	NET CARB (g)	GI VALUE	GI LEVEL	GL VALUE	GL LEVEL
Ham and Cheese Biscuits	1 biscuit, 60g	20	70	High	14	Med.
Hummingbird Cake	1 slice, 80g	37	74	High	27.4	High
Irish Soda Bread	1 slice, 45g	20	65	Med.	13	Med.
Italian Bread	1 slice, 30g	14	70	High	9.8	Low
Keto Bread	2 slice, 50g	4	10	Low	0.4	Low
Lemon Cake	1 slice, 100g	31	74	High	22.9	High
Lemon Cookies	1 cookie, 30g	14	73	High	10.2	Med.
Lemon Meringue Pie	1 slice, 125g	31	70	High	21.7	High
Lemon Mousse Tart	1 slice, 100g	22	76	High	16.7	Med.
Low-Carb Tortilla	1 med., 55g	6	30	Low	1.8	Low
Marble Cake	1 slice, 100g	36	74	High	26.6	High
Mille Crepe Cake	1 slice, 100g	33	74	High	24.4	High
Mississippi Mud Pie	1 slice, 100g	30	70	High	21	High
Mixed Berry Pie	1 slice, 100g	18	70	High	12.6	Med.
Molasses Cookies	1 cookie, 30g	17	73	High	12.4	Med.

BAKED FOODS & BREADS	SERVING SIZE	NET CARB (g)	GI VALUE	GI LEVEL	GL VALUE	GL LEVEL
Naan	1 piece, 60g	26	81	High	21.1	High
Oat Bread	1 slice, 25g	15	66	Med.	9.9	Low
Oatmeal Raisin Cookies	1 cookie, 30g	16	69	Med.	11	Med.
Orange Cake	1 slice, 80g	31	74	High	22.9	High
Panettone	1 slice, 50g	23	72	High	16.6	Med.
Peach Pie	1 slice, 125g	27	70	High	18.9	Med.
Peanut Butter Blossoms	1 cookie, 30g	13	76	High	9.9	Low
Peanut Butter Cookies	1 cookie, 30g	13	73	High	9.5	Low
Pecan Pie	1 slice, 125g	41	70	High	28.7	High
Pesto Biscuits	1 biscuit, 28g	15	70	High	10.5	Med.
Pita Bread	1 small pita, 35g	18	81	High	14.6	Med.
Pithivier	1 small, 90g	36	88	High	31.7	High
Pound Cake	1 slice, 100g	37	74	High	27.4	High
Pretzel	1 med., 60g	22	75	High	16.5	Med.
Puff Pastry	1 sheet, 79g	36	84	High	30.2	High

BAKED FOODS & BREADS	SERVING SIZE	NET CARB (g)	GI VALUE	GI LEVEL	GL VALUE	GL LEVEL
Pumpernickel Bread	1 slice, 25g	13	53	Low	6.9	Low
Pumpkin Biscuits	1 biscuit, 28g	15	70	High	10.5	Med.
Pumpkin Pie	1 slice, 125g	30	70	High	21	High
Quiche	1 slice, 100g	10	75	High	7.5	Low
Quinoa Bread	1 slice, 25g	13	30	Low	3.9	Low
Raspberry Tart	1 slice, 100g	15	76	High	11.4	Med.
Rhubarb Pie	1 slice, 125g	26	70	High	18.2	Med.
Rosemary Biscuits	1 biscuit, 38g	15	70	High	10.5	Med.
Rye Bread	1 slice, 25g	14	62	Med.	8.7	Low
Shortbread Cookies	1 cookie, 30g	11	73	High	8	Low
Simit	1 piece, 60g	22	78	High	17.2	Med.
Snickerdoodle Cookies	1 cookie , 30g	14	73	High	10.2	Med.
Sourdough Bread	1 slice, 25g	15	65	Med.	9.8	Low
Soy and Linseed Bread	1 slice, 25g	10	55	Low	5.5	Low
Spelt Bread	1 slice, 25g	16	53	Low	8.5	Low
Sponge Cake	1 slice, 100g	33	74	High	24.4	High

BAKED FOODS & BREADS	SERVING SIZE	NET CARB (g)	GI VALUE	GI LEVEL	GL VALUE	GL LEVEL
Strawberry ShortCake	1 slice, 100g	32	74	High	23.7	High
Strawberry Tart	1 biscuit, 50g	22	76	High	16.7	Med.
Strudel	1 slice, 100g	41	81	High	33.2	High
Sweet Potato Biscuits	1 cookie, 30g	16	70	High	11.2	Med.
Tiramisu	1 small, 60g	28	88	High	24.6	High
Tomato Tart	1 slice, 100g	30	76	High	22.8	High
Tres Leches Cake	1 slice, 100g	10	74	High	7.4	Low
Vanilla Cake	1 slice, 100g	42	74	High	31.1	High
Vol-au-vent	1 slice, 100g	34	82	High	27.9	High
Wheat Tortilla	1 med., 55g	18	70	High	12.6	Med.
Whole Grain Bread	1 slice, 25g	12	68	Med.	8.2	Low
Whole Grain Ciabatta	1 small, 25g	15	68	Med.	10.2	Med.
Whole Wheat Bread	1 slice, 30g	14	71	High	9.9	Low

3
LEGUMES AND LEGUMES FLOURS

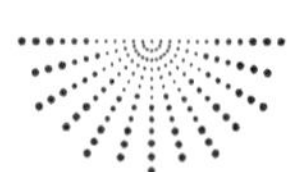

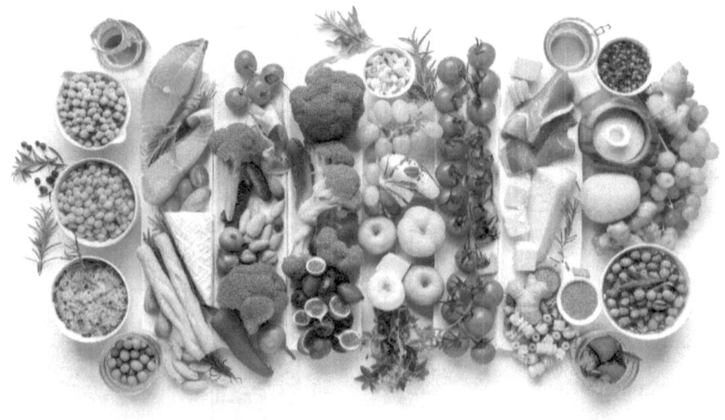

FOOD	SERVING SIZE	NET CARB (g)	GI VALUE	GI LEVEL	GL VALUE	GL LEVEL
Azuki Bean Flour	¼ cup, 30g	18.9	33	Low	6.2	Low
Baby lima beans	½ cup, 100g	13	32	Low	6	Low
Black Bean Flour	¼ cup, 30g	10.5	30	Low	3.2	Low
Black beans, mature seeds, soaked and cooked	½ cup, 100g	13	30	Low	5	Low
Black Eyed Pea Flour	¼ cup, 30g	18.9	42	Low	7.9	Low
Black turtle beans, mature, soaked cooked	½ cup, 100g	13	30	Low	5	Low
Black-eyed peas	½ cup, 100g	19	41	Low	8	Low
Broad Bean Flour (Fava Bean Flour)	¼ cup, 30g	17.4	79	High	13.7	Medium
Butter Bean Flour (Lima Bean Flour)	¼ cup, 30g	18	31	Low	5.6	Low
Cannellini Bean Flour	¼ cup, 30g	18	31	Low	5.6	Low
Cannellini beans, mature seeds, soaked and cooked	½ cup, 100g	13	31	Low	4	Low
Chia Sprout Powder	¼ cup, 30g	4	15	Low	0.6	Low
Chickpea Flour (Besan)	¼ cup, 30g	13.2	44	Low	5.8	Low

FOOD	SERVING SIZE	NET CARB (g)	GI VALUE	GI LEVEL	GL VALUE	GL LEVEL
Chickpeas	½ cup, 82g	13.5	28	Low	4	Low
Cowpeas	½ cup, 100g	18	29	Low	7	Low
Cowpeas, leafy tips, raw	1 cup, 36g	1	20	Low	1	Low
Cowpeas, young pods with seeds, raw	1 cup, 100g	8	40	Low	4	Low
Dragon's tongue beans, mature, soaked cooked	½ cup, 100g	5	31	Low	2	Low
Fava Bean Flour	¼ cup, 30g	17.4	79	High	13.7	Medium
Fava beans, mature seeds, soaked and cooked	½ cup, 100g	13	32	Low	7	Low
Flageolet beans, mature seeds, soaked and cooked	½ cup, 100g	14	31	Low	4	Low
French Green Lentil Flour	¼ cup, 30g	18	28	Low	5	Low
Garbanzo Bean Flour	¼ cup, 30g	17.4	28	Low	4.9	Low
Great Northern Bean Flour	¼ cup, 30g	18	36	Low	6.5	Low
Great Northern Beans, mature, soaked cooked	½ cup, 100g	15	31	Low	5	Low
Green Pea Flour	¼ cup, 30g	18	48	Low	8.6	Low
Green peas	½ cup, 100g	9	42	Low	4	Low

FOOD	SERVING SIZE	NET CARB (g)	GI VALUE	GI LEVEL	GL VALUE	GL LEVEL
Kidney Bean Flour	¼ cup, 30g	18	24	Low	4.3	Low
Kidney beans, mature seeds, soaked and cooked	½ cup, 100g	16	29	Low	7	Low
Lentil Flour	¼ cup, 30g	15	29	Low	4.4	Low
Lentil Sprout Powder	¼ cup, 30g	15	25	Low	3.8	Low
Lentils	½ cup, 100g	12	29	Low	5	Low
Lima bean flour	½ cup, 100g	19	32	Low	4	Low
Lima beans	½ cup, 100g	20	32	Low	8	Low
Moth Bean Flour	¼ cup, 30g	18.9	29	Low	5.5	Low
Mung Bean Flour	¼ cup, 30g	18.9	25	Low	4.7	Low
Mung Bean Sprout Powder	¼ cup, 30g	12	15	Low	1.8	Low
Mung beans, mature seeds, soaked and cooked	½ cup, 100g	12	32	Low	4	Low
Navy Bean Flour	¼ cup, 30g	18	38	Low	6.8	Low
Navy beans, mature seeds, soaked and cooked	½ cup, 100g	11	31	Low	3.5	Low
Pea Sprout Powder	¼ cup, 30g	14	15	Low	2.1	Low

FOOD	SERVING SIZE	NET CARB (g)	GI VALUE	GI LEVEL	GL VALUE	GL LEVEL
Pinto Bean Flour	¼ cup, 30g	18	39	Low	7	Low
Quinoa Sprout Powder	¼ cup, 30g	20	35	Low	7	Low
Red beans	½ cup, 100g	15	35	Low	5.3	Low
Red kidney beans	½ cup, 100g	13	40	Low	7	Low
Red Lentil Flour	¼ cup, 30g	18	26	Low	4.7	Low
Red lentils	½ cup, 100g	13	44	Low	8	Low
Soy Flour	¼ cup, 30g	6	15	Low	0.9	Low
Soybean Sprout Powder	¼ cup, 30g	8	15	Low	1.2	Low
Soybeans	½ cup, 100g	10	33	Low	6	Low
Split peas	½ cup, 100g	12	32	Low	5	Low
Sunflower Sprout Powder	¼ cup, 30g	8	15	Low	1.2	Low
White Bean Flour	¼ cup, 30g	18	31	Low	5.6	Low
White beans, mature seeds, soaked and cooked	½ cup, 100g	12	45	Low	7	Low
Yellow Split Pea Flour	¼ cup, 30g	18	35	Low	6.3	Low

4
BEVERAGES & DRINKS

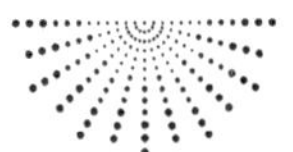

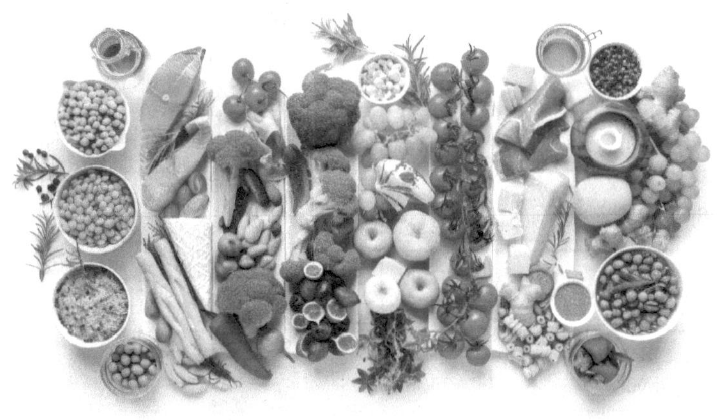

BEVERAGES & DRINKS	SERVING SIZE	NET CARB (g)	GI VALUE	GI LEVEL	GL VALUE	GL LEVEL
Apple Cider Vinegar - diluted as beverage-	1 cup, 240ml	0	0	Low	0	Low
Beer	1 cup, 240ml	8	50	Low	4	Low
Beer Birch	1 cup, 240ml	34	68	Med.	23.1	High
Beer light	1 cup, 240ml	4	50	Low	2	Low
Beer Root	1 cup, 240ml	30	63	Med.	18.9	Med.
Beet Kvass	1 cup, 240ml	10	60	Med.	6	Low
Cappuccino	1 cup, 240ml	8	50	Low	4	Low
Caramel Latte	1 cup, 240ml	25	50	Low	12.5	Med.
Caramel Macchiato	1 cup, 240ml	25	50	Low	12.5	Med.
Carbonated Lemonade	1 cup, 240ml	30	72	High	21.6	High
Carbonated Water with Natural Flavors	1 cup, 240ml	0	0	Low	0	Low
Coconut Water	1 cup, 240ml	9	35	Low	3.2	Low
Coffee Espresso	¼ cup, 60ml	0	0	Low	0	Low

BEVERAGES & DRINKS	SERVING SIZE	NET CARB (g)	GI VALUE	GI LEVEL	GL VALUE	GL LEVEL
Coffee Iced/Hot	1 cup, 240ml	0	0	Low	0	Low
Cola Soda regular	1 cup, 240ml	26	63	Med.	16.4	Med.
Cortado	4 fl oz, 120g	0	0	Low	0	Low
Cream Soda	1 cup, 240ml	30	71	High	21.3	High
Diet Cola	1 cup, 240ml	0	0	Low	0	Low
Diet Lemon-Lime Soda	1 cup, 240ml	0	0	Low	0	Low
Electrolyte Water	1 cup, 240ml	0	0	Low	0	Low
Energy Drink regular	1 cup, 240ml	28	72	High	20.2	High
Energy Drink sugar-free	1 cup, 240ml	0	0	Low	0	Low
Energy Shot	1 cup, 240ml	30	70	High	21	High
Frappuccino	1 cup, 240ml	50	50	Low	25	High
Fruit Punch	1 cup, 240ml	28	67	Med.	18.8	Med.
Ginger Ale	1 cup, 240ml	26	63	Med.	16.4	Med.
Grape Soda	1 cup, 240ml	40	63	Med.	25.2	High

BEVERAGES & DRINKS	SERVING SIZE	NET CARB (g)	GI VALUE	GI LEVEL	GL VALUE	GL LEVEL
Horchata	1 cup, 240ml	43	70	High	30.1	High
Hot Apple Toddy	1 cup, 240ml	10	0	Low	0	Low
Hot Chocolate	1 cup, 240ml	30	60	Med.	18	Med.
Iced Chai Tea Latte	1 cup, 240ml	25	50	Low	12.5	Med.
Isotonic Beverage	1 cup, 240ml	10	50	Low	5	Low
Kombucha	1 cup, 240ml	2	10	Low	0.2	Low
Kvass	1 cup, 240ml	7	40	Low	2.8	Low
Lactose-Free Protein Drink	1 cup, 240ml	3	30	Low	0.9	Low
Lassi Low-carb Drink	1 cup, 240ml	10	30	Low	3	Low
Latte Macchiato	1 cup, 240ml	10	40	Low	4	Low
Lemon-Lime Soda	1 cup, 240ml	26	63	Med.	16.4	Med.
Macchiato	1 cup, 240ml	10	40	Low	4	Low
Malt Drink	1 cup, 240ml	35	50	Low	17.5	Med.
Malted Milk	1 cup, 240ml	45	50	Low	22.5	High

BEVERAGES & DRINKS	SERVING SIZE	NET CARB (g)	GI VALUE	GI LEVEL	GL VALUE	GL LEVEL
Matcha Green Tea Iced/Hot	1 cup, 240ml	0	0	Low	0	Low
Milk Chocolate	1 cup, 240ml	23	60	Med.	13.8	Med.
Orange Soda Regular	1 cup, 240ml	28	72	High	20.2	High
Post-workout Recovery Drink	1 cup, 240ml	25	50	Low	12.5	Med.
Protein Shake	1 cup, 240ml	5	25	Low	1.3	Low
Protein Shake Whey Based	1 cup, 240ml	7	30	Low	2.1	Low
Pumpkin Spice Latte	1 cup, 240ml	52	70	High	36.4	High
Red Soda regular	1 cup, 240ml	31	63	Med.	19.5	High
Rice Wine	5 fl oz, 100g	3	10	Low	0.3	Low
Rum	1 fl oz, 30g	0	0	Low	0	Low
Sake	5 fl oz, 100g	1	20	Low	0.2	Low
Sarsaparilla	1 cup, 240ml	25	50	Low	12.5	Med.
Smoothie Chocolate Banana	1 cup, 240ml	68	45	Low	30.6	High
Sparkling Water	1 cup, 240ml	0	0	Low	0	Low

BEVERAGES & DRINKS	SERVING SIZE	NET CARB (g)	GI VALUE	GI LEVEL	GL VALUE	GL LEVEL
Stevia-Sweetened Soda	1 cup, 240ml	0	0	Low	0	Low
Tea Black/Green	1 cup, 240ml	0	0	Low	0	Low
Tea Bubble	1 cup, 240ml	60	70	High	42	High
Tea Chai /Chamomile /Ginger /Mint	1 cup, 240ml	0	0	Low	0	Low
Tea Herbal	1 cup, 240ml	0	0	Low	0	Low
Tea Thai Iced	1 cup, 240ml	25	50	Low	12.5	Med.
Tepache	1 cup, 240ml	25	55	Low	13.8	Med.
Tequila	1 fl oz, 30g	0	0	Low	0	Low
Tonic Water	1 cup, 240ml	25	50	Low	12.5	Med.
Vinegar -diluted as a beverage-	1 cup, 240ml	0	0	Low	0	Low
Vodka	1 fl oz, 30g	0	0	Low	0	Low
Whiskey	1 fl oz, 30g	0	0	Low	0	Low
Wine Mulled	5 fl oz, 148g	15	50	Low	7.5	Low
Wine red, white, rosé	5 fl oz, 148g	2.7	0	Low	0	Low

5

DAIRY PRODUCTS

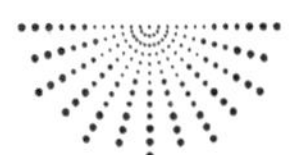

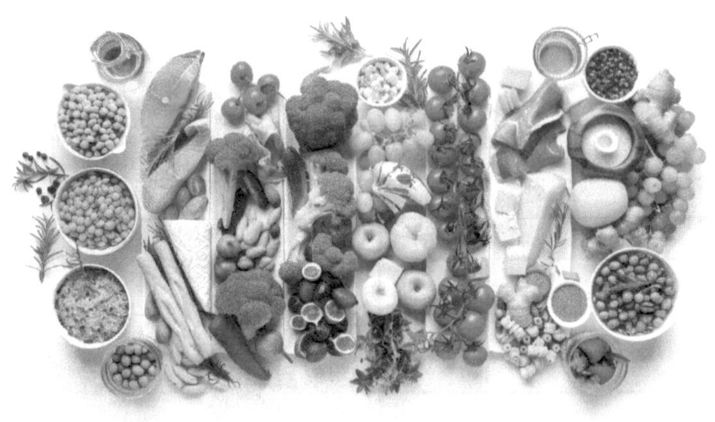

FOOD	SERVING SIZE	NET CARB (g)	GI VALUE	GI LEVEL	GL VALUE	GL LEVEL
American Cheese	1 oz, 28g	2	0	Low	0	Low
Blue cheese	1 oz, 28g	0.7	1-10	Low	0	Low
Brie Cheese	1 oz, 28g	1	0	Low	0	Low
Burrata	1 oz, 28g	1	1-10	Low	0.1	Low
Butter	1 tbsp, 14g	0	0	Low	0	Low
Buttermilk	1 cup, 245g	12	46	Low	5.5	Low
Camembert	1 oz, 28g	0.1	1-10	Low	0	Low
Cheddar	1 oz, 28g	0.4	1-10	Low	0.1	Low
Chèvre	1 oz, 28g	0.2	1-10	Low	0.1	Low
Colby Jack Cheese	1 oz, 28g	1	0	Low	0	Low
Comté	1 oz, 28g	0.4	1-10	Low	0.1	Low
Cottage Cheese	1 cup, 226g	6	10	Low	0.6	Low
Cream Cheese	1 oz, 28g	1	0	Low	0	Low
Creamer Dairy-based	1 tbsp, 15ml	5	47	Low	2.4	Low
Edam Cheese	1 oz, 28g	1	0	Low	0	Low
Emmental	1 oz, 28g	0.4	1-10	Low	0.1	Low
Farmer Cheese	1 cup, 226g	10	10	Low	1	Low
Feta	1 oz, 28g	1.2	1-10	Low	0.1	Low

FOOD	SERVING SIZE	NET CARB (g)	GI VALUE	GI LEVEL	GL VALUE	GL LEVEL
Fontina	1 oz, 28g	0.4	1-10	Low	0.1	Low
Ghee (Clarified Butter)	1 tbsp, 14g	0	0	Low	0	Low
Goat Cheese	1 oz, 28g	1	0	Low	0	Low
Gorgonzola	1 oz, 28g	0.3	1-10	Low	0.1	Low
Gouda Cheese	1 oz, 28g	1	0	Low	0	Low
Gruyere Cheese	1 oz, 28g	0	0	Low	0	Low
Halloumi	1 oz, 28g	1	1-10	Low	0.1	Low
Havarti Cheese	1 oz, 28g	1	0	Low	0	Low
Hot Mocha	1 cup, 240ml	30	50	Low	15	Med.
Iced Chai Tea Latte	1 cup, 240ml	25	50	Low	12.5	Med.
Kefir	1 cup, 240g	12	20	Low	2.4	Low
Labneh	1 oz, 28g	2	0	Low	0	Low
Limburger Cheese	1 oz, 28g	0	0	Low	0	Low
Manchego	1 oz, 28g	0	1-10	Low	0	Low
Mascarpone	1 oz, 28g	1	0	Low	0	Low
Milk Chocolate	1 cup, 240ml	23	60	Med.	13.8	Med.
Milk Lactose-free	1 cup, 244g	12	27-45	Low	5.4	Low

FOOD	SERVING SIZE	NET CARB (g)	GI VALUE	GI LEVEL	GL VALUE	GL LEVEL
Milk Skim	1 cup, 244g	12	27-45	Low	5.4	Low
Milk Whole	1 cup, 244g	12	27-45	Low	5.4	Low
Monterey Jack	1 oz, 28g	0.5	1-10	Low	0.1	Low
Monterey Jack Cheese	1 oz, 28g	1	0	Low	0	Low
Mozzarella	1 oz, 28g	0.6	1-10	Low	0.1	Low
Mozzarella Cheese	1 oz, 28g	1	0	Low	0	Low
Muenster	1 oz, 28g	0.3	1-10	Low	0.1	Low
Neufchâtel Cheese	1 oz, 28g	1	0	Low	0	Low
Panela Cheese	1 oz, 28g	0	0	Low	0	Low
Parmesan	1 oz, 28g	0.9	1-10	Low	0.1	Low
Pecorino Romano	1 oz, 28g	0.5	1-10	Low	0.1	Low
Pepper Jack	1 oz, 28g	0.5	1-10	Low	0.1	Low
Provolone Cheese	1 oz, 28g	1	0	Low	0	Low
Quark	1 cup, 225g	9	0	Low	0	Low
Queso Blanco	1 oz, 28g	0	0	Low	0	Low
Queso de Bola -Edam Cheese-	1 oz, 28g	0	0	Low	0	Low
Ricotta Cheese	1 cup, 246g	11	10	Low	1.1	Low
Ricotta Salata	1/4 cup, 62g	3	1-10	Low	0.3	Low

FOOD	SERVING SIZE	NET CARB (g)	GI VALUE	GI LEVEL	GL VALUE	GL LEVEL
Romano Cheese	1 oz, 28g	0	0	Low	0	Low
Sarsaparilla	1 cup, 240ml	25	50	Low	12.5	Med.
Sour Cream	1 cup, 230g	15	14	Low	2.1	Low
Stilton Cheese	1 oz, 28g	0.4	1-10	Low	0.1	Low
Swiss Cheese	1 oz, 28g	2	1-10	Low	0.2	Low
Taleggio	1 oz, 28g	0.1	1-10	Low	0.1	Low
Whipped Butter	1 tbsp, 14g	0	0	Low	0	Low
Whipped Cream	1 cup, 240g	10	0	Low	0	Low
Yogurt Greek Plain	1 cup, 245g	10	11	Low	1.1	Low
Yogurt Smoothie	1 cup, 240ml	30	50	Low	15	Med.

6

DAIRY ALTERNATIVES — PLANT-BASED OPTIONS

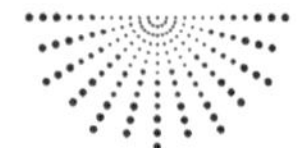

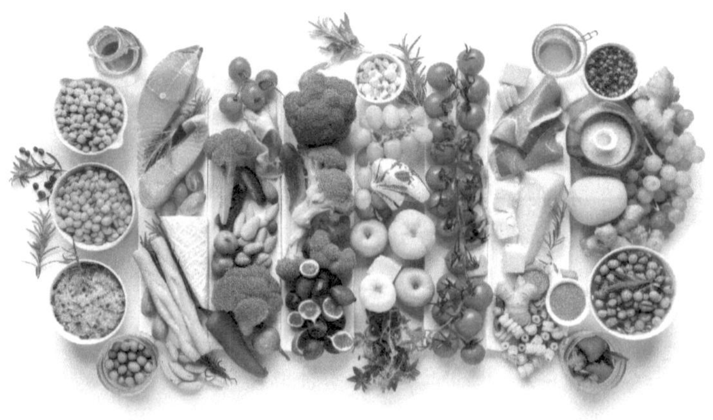

FOOD	SERVING SIZE	NET CARB (g)	GI VALUE	GI LEVEL	GL VALUE	GL LEVEL
Almond milk yogurt	1 cont., 150g	4	10	Low	0.4	Low
Almond milk	1 cup, 240 ml	2	30	Low	0.6	Low
Cashew milk yogurt	1 cont., 150g	7	10	Low	0.7	Low
Cashew milk	1 cup, 240 ml	4	30	Low	1.2	Low
Coconut milk yogurt	1 cont., 150g	15	50	Low	7.5	Low
Coconut Milk	1 cup, 240ml	21	50	Low	10.5	High
Creamer Non-dairy	1 tbsp, 15ml	4	34	Low	1.4	Low
Extra Firm Tofu	½ cup, 126g	2	15	Low	0.3	Low
Firm Tofu	½ cup, 126g	2	15	Low	0.3	Low
Flax milk	1 cup, 240 ml	1	10	Low	0.1	Low
Hazelnut milk	1 cup, 240 ml	19.9	50	Low	0.2	Low
Hemp milk	1 cup, 240 ml	2	20	Low	0.4	Low
Macadamia Milk	1 cup, 240ml	3	35	Low	1.1	Low

FOOD	SERVING SIZE	NET CARB (g)	GI VALUE	GI LEVEL	GL VALUE	GL LEVEL
Oat Milk	1 cup, 240ml	21	69	Med.	14.6	Med.
Pea milk	1 cup, 240 ml	2	34	Low	0.7	Low
Pistachio Milk	1 cup, 240ml	5	35	Low	1.8	Low
Post-workout Recovery Drink	1 cup, 240ml	25	50	Low	12.5	Med.
Pre-workout Energy Drink	1 cup, 240ml	30	65	Med.	19.5	Med.
Rice Milk	1 cup, 250ml	26	86	High	22.4	High
Quinoa Milk	1 cup, 240ml	8	54	Low	1.8	Low
Silken Tofu	½ cup, 126g	1	15	Low	0.2	Low
Soy Butter	1 tbsp, 14g	0	0	Low	0	Low
Soy Cheese	1 oz, 28g	0	14	Low	0	Low
Soy Cottage Cheese	1 cup, 240g	5	15	Low	0.8	Low
Soy Cream Cheese	1 oz, 28g	0	14	Low	0	Low
Soy Creamer	1 tbsp, 15ml	2	34	Low	0.7	Low
Soy Milk, Plain	Plain	4	34	Low	1.4	Low
Soy Milk	1 cup, 240ml	10	34	Low	3.4	Low

FOOD	SERVING SIZE	NET CARB (g)	GI VALUE	GI LEVEL	GL VALUE	GL LEVEL
Soy Protein Powder	1 scoop, 30g	2	25	Low	0.5	Low
Soy Ricotta Cheese	1 cup, 246g	4	15	Low	0.6	Low
Soy Sour Cream	1 tbsp, 14g	2	18	Low	0.4	Low
Soy Yogurt, Plain	1 cont., 150g	15	32	Low	4.8	Low
Soy-based Coffee Creamer	1 tbsp, 15ml	6	34	Low	0.7	Low
Soy-based Creamer	1 tbsp, 15ml	2	34	Low	0.7	Low
Soy-based Milkshake	1 cup, 240ml	15	34	Low	5.1	Low
Soy-based Whipped Cream	1 tbsp, 5g	15	0	Low	0	Low
Sports Drinks	1 cup, 240ml	0	60	Med.	18	Med.
Tempeh	1 cup, 166g	30	35	Low	3.5	Low
Tiger Nut Milk	1 cup, 240ml	25	65	Med.	15.6	Med.
Tofu	½ cup, 126g	24	15	Low	0.2	Low
Walnut Milk	1 cup, 240ml	1	25	Low	0.3	Low

7

DRESSINGS & OILS

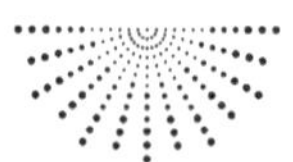

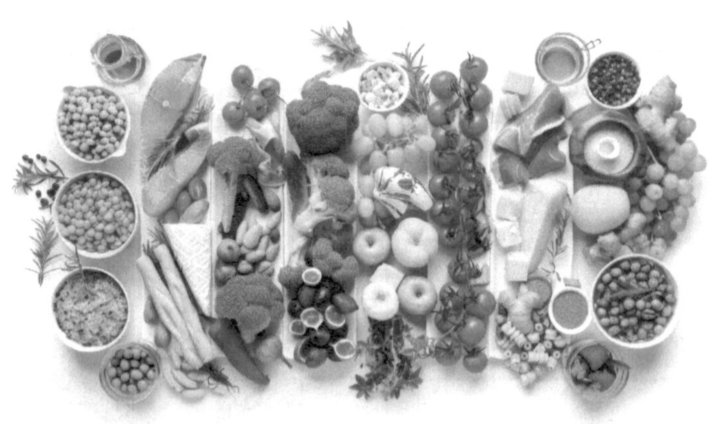

FOOD	SERVING SIZE	NET CARB (g)	GI VALUE	GI LEVEL	GL VALUE	GL LEVEL
Alfredo Sauce, Homemade	¼ cup, 62 g	1.6	27	Low	0.4	Low
Clarified Butter	1 tbsp, 15 g	0	0	L	0	Low
Cocktail sauce, Homemade	¼ cup, 62 g	18	38	Low	6.8	Low
Dressing, Blue or roquefort, Homemade	2 tbsp, 30 g	8.1	50	Low	4.1	Low
Dressing, Caesar, Homemade	¼ cup, 62 g	1.6	50	Low	0.8	Low
Dressing, Coleslaw, Homemade	¼ cup, 62 g	2.3	50	Low	1.2	Low
Dressing, Cream cheese, Homemade	2 tbsp, 30 g	1	50	Low	0.5	Low
Dressing, Feta Cheese, Homemade	¼ cup, 62 g	1.4	50	Low	0.7	Low
Dressing, French, Homemade	2 tbsp, 30 g	9	50	Low	4.5	Low
Dressing, Green Goddess, Homemade	2 tbsp, 30 g	2.4	50	Low	1.2	Low
Dressing, Honey mustard, Homemade	2 tbsp, 30 g	8.4	50	Low	4.2	Low
Dressing, Italian dressing, Homemade	2 tbsp, 30 g	2.2	50	Low	1.1	Low
Dressing, Korean, Homemade	¼ cup, 62 g	3.7	50	Low	1.9	Low

FOOD	SERVING SIZE	NET CARB (g)	GI VALUE	GI LEVEL	GL VALUE	GL LEVEL
Dressing, Mayonnaise-type salad, Homemade	2 tbsp, 30 g	6	50	Low	3	Low
Dressing, Milk, vinegar based, Homemade	2 tbsp, 30 g	1.9	50	Low	1	Low
Dressing, Peppercorn, Homemade	2 tbsp, 30 g	2	50	Low	1	Low
Dressing, Poppy seed, Homemade	2 tbsp, 30 g	6.2	50	Low	3.1	Low
Dressing, Russian, Homemade	2 tbsp, 30 g	9.6	50	Low	4.8	Low
Dressing, Salad, Vinegar based Homemade	2 tbsp, 30 g	2.8	50	Low	1.4	Low
Dressing, Sesame, Homemade	2 tbsp, 30 g	7.4	50	Low	3.7	Low
Dressing, Thousand Island, Homemade	2 tbsp, 30 g	2.9	50	Low	1.5	Low
Dressing, Yogurt, Homemade	2 tbsp, 30 g	1.9	50	Low	1	Low
Duck Fat	2 tbsp, 30 g	0	0	Low	0	Low
Mayonnaise, Homemade	2 tbsp, 30 g	2.4	50	Low	1.2	Low
Mayonnaise, Vegan tofu, Homemade	2 tbsp, 30 g	0.6	50	Low	0.3	Low
Mustard greens (mean value)	2 tbsp, 30 g	0.5	32	Low	0.2	Low
Oil, Avocado	2 tbsp, 30 g	0	0	Low	0	Low

FOOD	SERVING SIZE	NET CARB (g)	GI VALUE	GI LEVEL	GL VALUE	GL LEVEL
Oil, Canola	2 tbsp, 30 g	0	0	Low	0	Low
Oil, Coconut	2 tbsp, 30 g	0	0	Low	0	Low
Oil, Corn	2 tbsp, 30 g	0	0	Low	0	Low
Oil, Extra-virgin olive	2 tbsp, 30 g	0	0	Low	0	Low
Oil, Flaxseed	2 tbsp, 30 g	0	0	Low	0	Low
Oil, Grapeseed	2 tbsp, 30 g	0	0	Low	0	Low
Oil, Hazelnut	2 tbsp, 30 g	0	0	Low	0	Low
Oil, Hemp seed	2 tbsp, 30 g	0	0	Low	0	Low
Oil, Peanut	2 tbsp, 30 g	0	0	Low	0	Low
Oil, Rice Bran	2 tbsp, 30 g	0	0	Low	0	Low
Oil, Sesame	2 tbsp, 30 g	0	0	Low	0	Low
Oil, Sunflower	2 tbsp, 30 g	0	0	Low	0	Low
Oil, Walnut	2 tbsp, 30 g	0	0	Low	0	Low

8

FRUITS

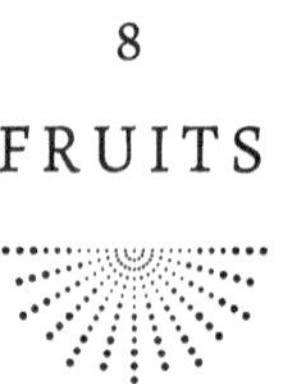

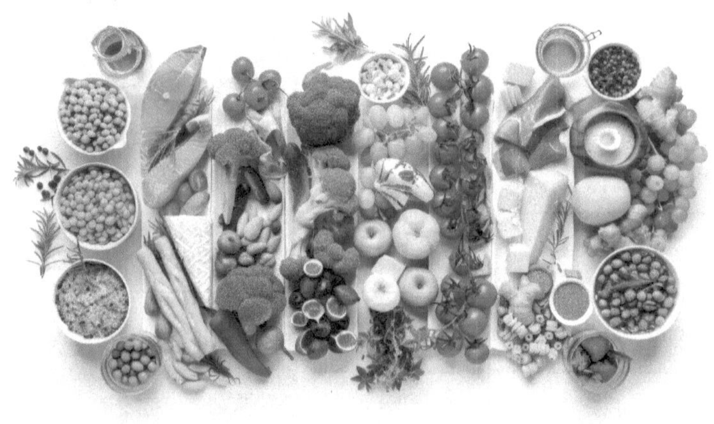

FOOD	SERVING SIZE	NET CARB (g)	GI VALUE	GI LEVEL	GL VALUE	GL LEVEL
Abiyuch	½ cup, 64g	16	45	Low	7.2	Low
Acai	½ cup, 100g	5	40	Low	2	Low
Acerola	1 cup, 98g	8	25	Low	2	Low
Ackee	½ cup, 100g	8	50	Low	4	Low
Apple	1 med., 182g	21	36	Low	5	Low
Apple Star	1 fruit, 138g	6	35	Low	3	Low
Apple Velvet	1 fruit, 166g	9	35	Low	3	Low
Apples Golden Delicious	1 med., 174g	17	40	Low	6	Low
Apples Granny Smith	1 med., 170g	14	35	Low	5	Low
Apricot Plum	1 fruit, 50g	7	34	Low	2	Low
Asian Pears	1 med., 166g	17	35	Low	6	Low
Avocados	½ fruit, 100g	3	20	Low	1	Low
Banana Baked	1 small, 81g	24	88	High	20.3	High
Banana extra ripe raw	1 small, 81g	22	85	High	18.7	med.

FOOD	SERVING SIZE	NET CARB (g)	GI VALUE	GI LEVEL	GL VALUE	GL LEVEL
Banana ripe raw	1 small , 81g	23	75	High	16.5	med.
Banana Unripe	1 small, 81g	19	53	Low	10	Low
Black Sapote	½ cup, 50g	9	35	Low	3	Low
Blackberries	1 cup, 144g	10	30	Low	3	Low
Blackberry	½ cup, 72g	7	25	Low	2	Low
Blueberry	½ cup, 75g	10	40	Low	4	Low
Boysenberry	½ cup, 75g	8	30	Low	3	Low
Breadfruit	½ cup, 60g	12	60	med.	6	Low
Cantaloupe	½ cup, 89g	7	60	med.	4	Low
Cape Gooseberry	½ cup, 50g	7	40	Low	3	Low
Carissa	1 cup, 132g	18	40	Low	7	Low
Cherimoya	½ fruit, 85g	9	35	Low	3	Low
Cherry	½ cup, 76g	10	22	Low	3	Low
Chokeberry	½ cup, 60g	6	35	Low	2	Low
Clementine	1 fruit, 74g	9	35	Low	3	Low
Cloudberry	½ cup, 60g	5	25	Low	2	Low
Coconut	½ cup, 40g	5	45	Low	2	Low
Cornelian Cherry	½ cup, 75g	6	30	Low	2	Low
Cranberry	½ cup, 50g	6	45	Low	3	Low
Currant	½ cup, 56g	8	25	Low	2	Low

FOOD	SERVING SIZE	NET CARB (g)	GI VALUE	GI LEVEL	GL VALUE	GL LEVEL
Dates	¼ cup, 40g	28	70	Low	21	High
Durian	½ cup, 100g	13	45	Low	6	Low
Feijoa	1 fruit, 50g	6	35	Low	2	Low
Fig Fresh	1 med., 50g	14	60	med.	8	Low
Figs dried	¼ cup, 40g	24	61	med.	15	med.
Finger Lime	1 fruit, 10g	1	30	Low	0	Low
Goji Berries Dried	¼ cup, 28g	17	40	Low	7.5	Low
Goldenberry	½ cup, 50g	6	35	Low	3	Low
Gooseberry	½ cup, 75g	8	25	Low	2	Low
Grape	½ cup, 75g	13	46	Low	5	Low
Grapefruit	1 med., 154g	13	30	Low	4	Low
Guanabana	½ cup, 100g	10	40	Low	4	Low
Guava	1 med., 55g	4	20	Low	1	Low
Hala Fruit	¼ cup, 25g	2	35	Low	1	Low
Jackfruit	½ cup, 100g	16	50	Low	8	Low
Jambul	½ cup, 75g	5	30	Low	2	Low
Jujube	1 fruit, 15g	6	50	Low	3	Low

FOOD	SERVING SIZE	NET CARB (g)	GI VALUE	GI LEVEL	GL VALUE	GL LEVEL
Kiwano	½ fruit, 100g	7	35	Low	2	Low
Kiwi	1 fruit, 69g	9	50	Low	5	Low
Kumquat	5 fruits , 50g	6	30	Low	3	Low
Langsat	½ cup, 75g	8	40	Low	3	Low
Lemon	1 fruit, 58g	3	20	Low	1	Low
Lime	1 fruit, 44g	3	20	Low	1	Low
Limequat	1 fruit, 20g	2	30	Low	1	Low
Litchis	1 cup, 190g	25	54	Low	14	med.
Loganberries	1 cup, 180g	9	30	Low	3	Low
Longan	½ cup, 50g	10	50	Low	5	Low
Loquat	½ cup, 75g	5	35	Low	2	Low
Lychee	½ cup, 75g	12	54	Low	7.1	Low
Mango	½ cup, 83g	15	54	Low	8	Low
Mangosteen	1 fruit, 75g	6	45	Low	3	Low
Melon	1 cup, 177g	12	65	med.	5	Low
Melon Honeydew	½ cup, 85g	8	60	med.	4	Low
Melon Santa Claus	1 cup, 177g	13	60	med.	6	Low
Miracle Fruit	1 fruit, 5g	1	30	Low	0	Low
Mulberry	½ cup, 70g	6	25	Low	3	Low
Nance	1 cup, 120g	20	45	Low	10	Low

FOOD	SERVING SIZE	NET CARB (g)	GI VALUE	GI LEVEL	GL VALUE	GL LEVEL
Nectarines	1 med., 142g	15	40	Low	6	Low
Olive	5 large, 25g	1	15	Low	0	Low
Orange	1 med., 131g	12	40	Low	4	Low
Papaya	1 cup, 145g	11	60	med.	6	Low
Passion Fruit	1 fruit, 18g	2	30	Low	1	Low
Peach	1 med., 150g	10	40	Low	4	Low
Pear	1 med., 178g	21	38	Low	5	Low
Persimmon	1 fruit, 25g	6	50	Low	3	Low
Pineapple	½ cup, 82g	10	59	med.	7	Low
Pitanga	1 cup, 140g	14	40	Low	7	Low
Plantains Cooked	½ cup, 100g	32	54	Low	17.6	med.
Plum	1 fruit, 66g	6	40	Low	2	Low
Plum Japanese	1 fruit, 40g	4	40	Low	2	Low
Pomegranate	½ cup, 87g	12	53	Low	6	Low
Pomelo	½ fruit, 154g	9	30	Low	3	Low
Prunes	¼ cup, 40g	18	29	Low	10	Low
Quince	1 fruit, 92g	6	34	Low	2	Low

FOOD	SERVING SIZE	NET CARB (g)	GI VALUE	GI LEVEL	GL VALUE	GL LEVEL
Raisin	¼ cup, 40g	31	66	med.	20.5	High
Raspberry	½ cup, 62g	3	32	Low	1	Low
Red Banana	1 med., 100g	18	45	Low	7	Low
Redcurrant	½ cup, 56g	5	25	Low	2	Low
Rhubarb	1 cup, 122g	3	15	Low	1	Low
Sapodilla	1 fruit, 150g	14	45	Low	6	Low
Soursop	1 cup, 225g	15	45	Low	6	Low
Star Fruit	1 fruit, 91g	4	25	Low	1	Low
Strawberry	½ cup, 72g	4	32	Low	1	Low
Tamarind	1 oz, 28g	6	40	Low	3	Low
Tangelo	1 fruit, 109g	10	42	Low	4	Low
Tangerine	1 fruit, 84g	9	40	Low	3	Low
Watermelon	1 cup, 152g	11	72	High	5	Low
White Currant	½ cup, 56g	5	25	Low	2	Low
White Sapote	1 fruit, 170g	6	30	Low	2	Low
Yellow Passion Fruit	1 fruit, 18g	2	30	Low	1	Low
Yellow Watermelon	1 cup, 152g	11	72	High	5	Low
Zante Currant	¼ cup, 40g	17	60	med.	10	Low
Ziziphus Fruit	5 fruit, 50g	15	35	Low	5.2	Low

9
FRUIT PRODUCTS

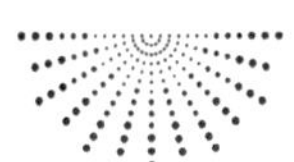

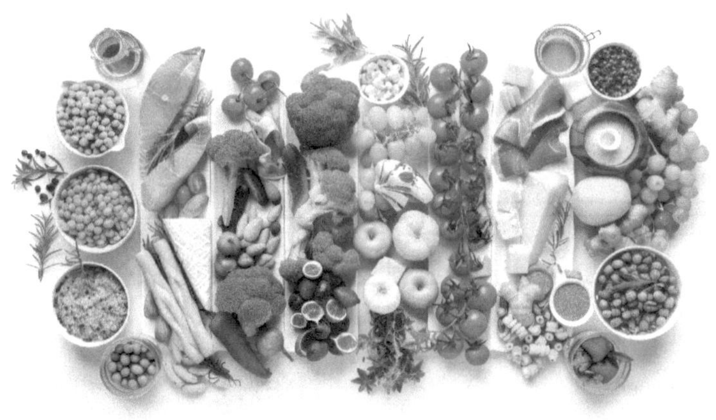

FOOD	SERVING SIZE	NET CARB (g)	GI VALUE	GI LEVEL	GL VALUE	GL LEVEL
Acerola Juice	½ cup, 120ml	6	40	Low	2.4	Low
Apple Baked Unsweetened	1 cup, 125g	23	40	Low	8	Low
Apple Butter	1 tbsp, 20g	10	45	Low	6	Low
Apple Chips	1 cup, 30g	22	50	Low	10	Low
Apple Juice, 100% fruit	½ cup, 120ml	14	45	Low	6.3	Low
Apple Pickled	½ cup, 75g	12	35	Low	4	Low
Applesauce	¼ cup, 61g	12.5	40	Low	5	Low
Apricot	1 fruit, 35g	4	34	Low	2	Low
Apricot Jam Unsweetened	1 tbsp, 20g	13	54	Low	8	Low
Apricot Juice Concentrate	¼ cup, 60g	12	40	Low	6	Low
Apricots Canned Light Syrup Drained	½ cup, 122g	14	45	Low	7	Low
Blackberries canned Light Syrup Drained	½ cup, 122g	8	25	Low	3	Low
Blackberry Jam Homemade	1 tbsp, 20g	13	54	Low	8	Low
Blackcurrant Juice Concentrate	¼ cup, 60g	0	20	Low	0	Low
Blueberries Canned Light Syrup Drained	1 cup, 230g	23	45	Low	10	Low

FOOD	SERVING SIZE	NET CARB (g)	GI VALUE	GI LEVEL	GL VALUE	GL LEVEL
Blueberry Jam Homemade	1 tbsp, 20g	13	54	Low	8	Low
Blueberry Juice, 100% fruit	½ cup, 120ml	14	40	Low	5.8	Low
Carrot Juice, 100% fruit	½ cup, 120ml	9.5	43	Low	4.1	Low
Cherries Canned Light Syrup Drained	½ cup, 122g	18	60	med.	9	Low
Cherry Juice, 100% fruit	½ cup, 120ml	14	50	Low	7	Low
Cherry Preserves	1 tbsp, 20g	13	54	Low	8	Low
Cranberry Juice, 100% fruit	½ cup, 120ml	15	52	Low	7.5	Low
Cranberry Sauce Homemade	1 tbsp, 20g	13	54	Low	8	Low
Desert Lime	1 fruit, 30g	3	30	Low	1	Low
Dried Apple	¼ cup, 28g	16	44	Low	10	Low
Dried Apricots Unsweetened	¼ cup, 32g	18	32	Low	12	med.
Dried Banana Unsweetened	¼ cup, 30g	22	54	Low	14	med.
Dried Blueberries Unsweetened	¼ cup, 40g	26	53	Low	14	med.
Dried Cherries Unsweetened	¼ cup, 40g	30	54	Low	16	med.
Dried Coconut	¼ cup, 20g	7	40	Low	3	Low

FOOD	SERVING SIZE	NET CARB (g)	GI VALUE	GI LEVEL	GL VALUE	GL LEVEL
Dried Cranberries Unsweetened	¼ cup, 40g	28	64	med.	18	med.
Dried Currants Unsweetened	¼ cup, 40g	30	56	med.	17	med.
Dried Custard Apple Unsweetened	¼ cup, 30g	22	48	Low	13	med.
Dried Dragon Fruit	¼ cup, 28g	15	57	med.	9	Low
Dried Goji Berries	¼ cup, 28g	14	29	Low	7	Low
Dried Guava	¼ cup, 30g	18	45	Low	10	Low
Dried Kiwi Unsweetened	¼ cup, 30g	19	54	Low	11	med.
Dried Longan Unsweetened	¼ cup, 32g	28	54	Low	15	med.
Dried Lychee Unsweetened	¼ cup, 30g	22	52	Low	13	med.
Dried Mango Unsweetened	¼ cup, 30g	22	57	med.	12	med.
Dried Papaya Unsweetened	¼ cup, 30g	25	60	med.	15	med.
Dried Peach	¼ cup, 36g	20	35	Low	10	Low
Dried Pear Unsweetened	¼ cup, 40g	24	43	Low	12	med.
Dried Persimmon	¼ cup, 32g	24	53	Low	15	med.
Dried Pineapple Unsweetened	¼ cup, 35g	28	58	med.	16	med.
Dried Raspberries	¼ cup, 30g	16	40	Low	8	Low

FOOD	SERVING SIZE	NET CARB (g)	GI VALUE	GI LEVEL	GL VALUE	GL LEVEL
Dried Sapodilla Unsweetened	¼ cup, 30g	20	50	Low	12	med.
Dried Strawberries	¼ cup, 30g	18	50	Low	10	Low
Fig Preserves	1 tbsp, 20g	13	54	Low	8	Low
Grape Jelly Homemade	1 tbsp, 20g	13	54	Low	8	Low
Grape Juice Concentrate	¼ cup, 60g	15	70	High	12	med.
Grapefruit Juice, 100% fruit	½ cup, 120ml	11	48	Low	5	Low
Grapefruit segments Canned Light Syrup Drained	½ cup, 122g	10	25	Low	3	Low
Guava Canned Light Syrup Drained	½ cup, 122g	10	50	Low	5	Low
Guava Juice, 100% fruit	½ cup, 120ml	10	33	Low	3.3	Low
Guava Nectar Canned Light	1 cup, 240g	30	45	Low	15	med.
Guava Sauce Cooked	1 cup, 250g	28	45	Low	14	med.
Lemon Curd Homemade	1 tbsp, 20g	13	54	Low	8	Low
Lemon Juice, 100% fruit	½ cup, 120ml	10.5	20	Low	2	Low
Lime Juice Concentrate	1 tbsp, 15g	1	20	Low	0.2	Low
Mango Canned Light Syrup Drained	½ cup, 122g	16	50	Low	8	Low
Mango Jam	1 tbsp, 20g	13	54	Low	8	Low

FOOD	SERVING SIZE	NET CARB (g)	GI VALUE	GI LEVEL	GL VALUE	GL LEVEL
Mango Juice, 100% fruit	½ cup, 120ml	15	41	Low	6.2	Low
Mango Pickled	¼ cup, 60g	12	45	Low	6	Low
Mixed Berry Jam	1 tbsp, 20g	13	54	Low	8	Low
Okra Pickled	1 cup, 160g	3	20	Low	1	Low
Orange Juice	½ cup, 120ml	13	50	Low	6.5	Low
Orange Marmalade Homemade	1 tbsp, 20g	13	54	Low	8	Low
Oranges Mandarin Canned Light Syrup Drained	½ cup, 122g	13	45	Low	6	Low
Papaya Canned Light Syrup Drained	½ cup, 122g	14	60	med.	7	Low
Passionfruit Juice, 100% fruit	½ cup, 120ml	7	30	Low	2.1	Low
Peach Juice, 100% fruit	½ cup, 120ml	14	42	Low	6	Low
Peach Pickled	½ cup, 130g	16	45	Low	8	Low
Peach Preserves Homemade	1 tbsp, 20g	13	54	Low	8	Low
Peaches Canned Light Syrup Drained	½ cup, 122g	16	45	Low	8	Low
Pear Juice, 100% fruit	½ cup, 120ml	14	44	Low	5.5	Low

FOOD	SERVING SIZE	NET CARB (g)	GI VALUE	GI LEVEL	GL VALUE	GL LEVEL
Pears Canned Extra Light Syrup	½ cup, 122g	11	45	Low	5.5	Low
Pears Canned Light Syrup Drained	½ cup, 122g	15	43	Low	7	Low
Peppers Pickled	1 cup, 150g	3	20	Low	1	Low
Pineapple Canned Extra Light Syrup	½ cup, 122g	15	54	Low	7.5	Low
Pineapple Frozen Chunks Unsweetened	½ cup, 82g	21	58	med.	12.1	med.
Pineapple Juice, 100% fruit	½ cup, 120ml	14	46	Low	6.5	Low
Pineapple Preserves	1 tbsp, 20g	14	55	Low	8	Low
Plum Jam	1 tbsp, 20g	13	54	Low	8	Low
Plum Pickled	1 cup, 150g	12	35	Low	6	Low
Plums Canned Extra Purple Light Syrup	½ cup, 122g	15	45	Low	6.7	Low
Plums Canned Light Syrup Drained	½ cup, 122g	12	40	Low	6	Low
Pomegranate Juice, 100% fruit	½ cup, 120ml	17	53	Low	9	Low
Pomegranate Juice Concentrate	¼ cup, 60g	12	35	Low	8	Low
Prune Puree	¼ cup, 60g	24	45	Low	12	med.
Prune Whip	½ cup, 125g	28	45	Low	14	med.

FOOD	SERVING SIZE	NET CARB (g)	GI VALUE	GI LEVEL	GL VALUE	GL LEVEL
Purple Passion Fruit Juice, 100% fruit	½ cup, 120ml	10	35	Low	5	Low
Quince Jelly	1 tbsp, 20g	13	54	Low	8	Low
Raspberries Canned Light Syrup Drained	½ cup, 122g	9	32	Low	3	Low
Raspberry Jam	1 tbsp, 20g	13	54	Low	8	Low
Raspberry Juice, 100% fruit	¼ cup, 60g	10	40	Low	5	Low
Red Currant Jelly	1 tbsp, 20g	13	54	Low	8	Low
Strawberry Jam	1 tbsp, 20g	13	54	Low	8	Low
Strawberry Juice, 100% fruit	¼ cup, 60g	10	40	Low	5	Low
Tomato Juice, 100% fruit	1 cup, 240ml	10	38	Low	3.8	Low
Tsukemono Japanese Pickles	1 cup, 150g	4	20	Low	2	Low
Turnip Pickled	1 cup, 150g	3	20	Low	1	Low
Watermelon Juice, 100% fruit	½ cup, 120ml	9	72	High	7.2	Low

10
GRAINS, CEREALS, PASTA & RICE

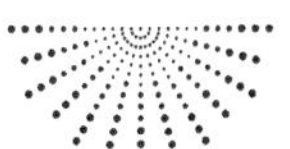

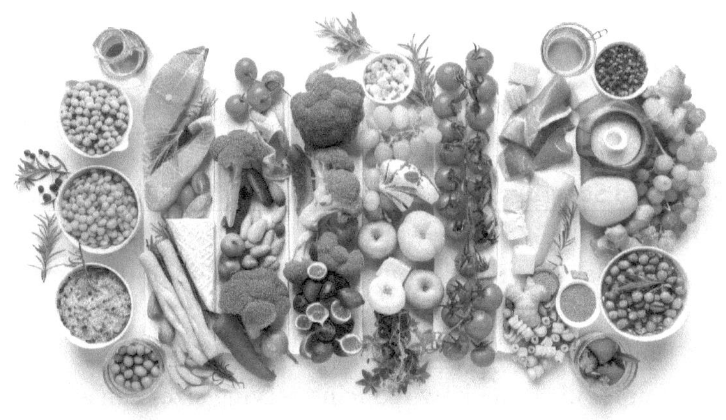

CARBOHYDRATE CONSIDERATIONS IN THE LOW GL DIABETES DIET

Grains and cereals play a significant role in the Low GL Diabetes Diet, and an analysis of their nutritional values is crucial for effective dietary management. Despite their integral role, most grains, cereals, and their products exhibit high Glycemic Load (GL) due to their high net carbohydrate content per standard serving size. The serving sizes listed are standard and not tailored to the guidelines of the Low GL Diabetes Diet, which stipulate that one serving should contain no more than 15 grams of net carbohydrates.

To align with these guidelines, consider the following examples of grains with low Glycemic Index (GI) values and calculate the portion sizes to fit the 15-gram net carb limit (see the following table for more details)

Whole Wheat Pasta:

- **GI Value**: Low (45)
- **Standard Serving Size**: 1 cup cooked (140g) yielding 49g net carbs.
- **Adjusted Serving Size**: Roughly ⅓ cup cooked to meet the 15g net carb requirement, minimizing the GL impact.

Egg Noodles:

- **GI Value**: Low (40)
- **Standard Serving Size**: 1 cup cooked (140g) yielding 50g net carbs.
- **Adjusted Serving Size**: About ⅓ cup cooked to fit the 15g net carb guideline, enhancing glycemic control.

These examples illustrate how reducing serving sizes can adapt high-carb foods to fit a low GL dietary pattern, emphasizing that even small amounts of certain grains can contribute effectively to a diabetes-friendly diet without causing significant spikes in blood glucose.

FOOD	SERVING SIZE	NET CARB (g)	GI VALUE	GI LEVEL	GL VALUE	GL LEVEL
Amaranth	1 cup cooked (246g)	20g	35	Low	7	Low
Arrowroot Flour	1 cup (120g)	105g	69	Med.	33	High
Barley	1 cup cooked (157g)	32g	28	Low	9	Low
Barley Flour or Meal	1 cup (128g)	76g	55	Low	24	High
Barley Hulled	1 cup cooked (157g)	41g	30	Low	11	Med.
Barley Malt Flour	1 cup (122g)	84g	65	Med.	36	High
Bucatini	1 cup cooked (140g)	49g	45	Low	22	High
Buckwheat	1 cup cooked (168g)	33g	55	Low	15	Med.
Buckwheat	1 cup cooked (168g)	33g	55	Low	17	Med.
Buckwheat Flour Whole-Groat	1 cup (120g)	72g	50	Low	26	High
Buckwheat Groats	1 cup cooked (168g)	29g	45	Low	13	Med.
Buckwheat Porridge	1 cup cooked (168g)	23g	65	Med.	14	Med.
Bulgur	1 cup cooked (182g)	26g	46	Low	12	Med.
Congee	1 cup cooked (250g)	45g	76	High	30	High
Corn Bran Crude	1 cup (60g)	19g	45	Low	9	Low
Corn Flour Masa White	1 cup (114g)	77g	65	Med.	42	High

FOOD	SERVING SIZE	NET CARB (g)	GI VALUE	GI LEVEL	GL VALUE	GL LEVEL
Corn Flour Whole-Grain Blue	1 cup (128g)	76g	55	Low	34	High
Corn Flour Whole-Grain Yellow	1 cup (128g)	76g	55	Low	34	High
Corn Flour Degermed	1 cup (125g)	71g	55	Low	31	High
Corn Grain	1 cup cooked (164g)	45g	60	Med.	27	High
Cornmeal	1/4 cup dry (30g)	20g	69	Med.	15	Med.
Cornmeal Degermed	1 cup (138g)	75g	55	Low	32	High
Cornstarch	1 cup (128g)	107g	90	High	43	High
Couscous	1 cup cooked (157g)	36g	65	Med.	22	High
Cream of Wheat	1 cup cooked (244g)	26g	85	High	19	Med.
Eggplant Lasagna	1 cup (240g))	20g	50	Low	10	Low
Farina	1 cup cooked (242g)	26g	80	High	19	Med.
Farro	1 cup cooked (169g)	45g	40	Low	18	Med.
Four Cheese Lasagna	1 cup (240g))	20g	50	Low	8	Low
Freekeh	1 cup cooked (162g)	28g	43	Low	12	Med.
Garlic and Herb Penne	2 ounces (56g)	41g	50	Low	18	Med.
Gluten-Free Penne	2 ounces (56g)	43g	40	Low	10	Low
Grits	1 cup cooked (242g)	28g	80	High	15	Med.

FOOD	SERVING SIZE	NET CARB (g)	GI VALUE	GI LEVEL	GL VALUE	GL LEVEL
Hulled Barley	1 cup cooked (157g)	32g	28	Low	9	Low
Japanese Somen	1 cup (145g)	37g	50	Low	17	Med.
Kamut	1 cup cooked (172g)	45g	45	Low	20	High
Kamut Pasta	1 cup cooked (140g)	43g	50	Low	20	High
Mexican Lasagna	1 cup (240g))	35g	50	Low	15	Med.
Millet Flour	1 cup (120g)	87g	75	High	39	High
Millet Porridge	1 cup cooked (200g)	24g	70	High	14	Med.
Millet Raw	1 cup (200g)	82g	76	High	36	High
Multigrain Penne	2 ounces (56g)	41g	50	Low	11	Med.
Mushroom Lasagna	1 cup (240g))	33g	50	Low	13	Med.
Noodles, Brown Rice	1 cup cooked (180g)	40g	65	Med.	24	High
Noodles, Buckwheat	1 cup cooked (114g)	42g	45	Low	19	Med.
Noodles, Chow Mein	1 cup cooked (140g)	49g	45	Low	22	High
Noodles, Egg	1 cup cooked (140g)	50g	40	Low	20	High
Noodles, Gluten Free Corn	1 cup (200g)	42g	65	Med.	27	High
Noodles, Japanese Soba	1 cup cooked (140g)	44g	60	Med.	25	High
Noodles, Ramen	1 cup cooked (140g)	48g	46	Low	22	High

FOOD	SERVING SIZE	NET CARB (g)	GI VALUE	GI LEVEL	GL VALUE	GL LEVEL
Oat Bran	1 cup (94g)	44g	60	Med.	21	High
Oat Flour Partially Debranned	1 cup (120g)	69g	60	Med.	31	High
Oat Rolled	1 cup cooked (234g)	27g	57	Med.	15.4	Med.
Oats Steel-Cut	1 cup cooked (240g)	27g	54	Low	15	Med.
Pearled Barley	1 cup (157g)	41g	30	Low	11	Med.
Penne Ziti	2 ounces (56g)	41g	50	Low	18	Med.
Pesto Lasagna	1 cup (240g))	30g	50	Low	10	Low
Polenta	1 cup cooked (128g)	24g	85	High	18	Med.
Quinoa	1 cup cooked (185g)	34g	53	Low	10	Low
Quinoa Porridge	1 cup cooked (185g)	23g	65	Med.	13	Med.
Rice, Arborio	1 cup cooked (200g)	50g	70	High	33	High
Rice, Basmati	1 cup cooked (160g)	44g	65	Med.	24	High
Rice, Bhutanese Red	1 cup cooked (185g)	42g	55	Low	21	High
Rice, Black	1 cup cooked (186g)	45g	48	Low	16	Med.
Rice, Brown	1 cup cooked (195g)	42g	55	Low	22	High
Rice, Brown Basmati	1 cup cooked (195g)	45g	58	Med.	21	High

FOOD	SERVING SIZE	NET CARB (g)	GI VALUE	GI LEVEL	GL VALUE	GL LEVEL
Rice, Brown Jasmine	1 cup cooked (195g)	42g	60	Med.	22	High
Rice, Calrose	1 cup cooked (160g)	40g	75	High	28	High
Rice, Carnaroli	1 cup cooked (200g)	50g	70	High	33	High
Rice, Cream of	1 cup cooked (240g)	27g	85	High	20	High
Rice, Forbidden	1 cup cooked (186g)	45g	48	Low	16	Med.
Rice, Glutinous	1 cup cooked (174g)	42g	91	High	37	High
Rice, Jasmine	1 cup cooked (158g)	45g	74	High	29	High
Rice, Noodles	1 cup cooked (170g)	40g	55	Low	22	High
Rice, Red	1 cup cooked (185g)	42g	55	Low	21	High
Rice, Sushi	1 cup cooked (150g)	40g	80	High	30	High
Rice, Wehani	1 cup cooked (185g)	42g	55	Low	21	High
Rice, White	1 cup cooked (158g)	45g	78	High	29	High
Rice, Wild	1 cup cooked (164g)	32g	55	Low	16	Med.
Rye	1 slice of bread (32g)	14g	62	Med.	10	Low
Rye Flour Dark	1 cup (102g)	63g	45	Low	21	High
Rye Flour Light	1 cup (102g)	57g	45	Low	19	Med.

FOOD	SERVING SIZE	NET CARB (g)	GI VALUE	GI LEVEL	GL VALUE	GL LEVEL
Rye Flour Medium	1 cup (102g)	60g	45	Low	20	High
Rye Grain	1 cup cooked (174g)	31g	50	Low	14	Med.
Seafood Lasagna	1 cup (240g))	25g	50	Low	10	Low
Semolina	1 cup (167g)	97g	60	Med.	32	High
Semolina Porridge	1 cup cooked (167g)	22g	65	Med.	13	Med.
Soba	1 cup cooked (114g)	42g	45	Low	19	Med.
Sorghum	1 cup cooked (192g)	29g	65	Med.	19	Med.
Sorghum Flour Refined	1 cup (125g)	83g	70	High	33	High
Sorghum Grain	1 cup cooked (192g)	51g	69	Med.	30	High
Spaghetti Spinach Cooked	1 cup (140g)	49g	45	Med.	22	High
Spaghetti Spinach Dry	1 cup (100g)	70g	45	Low	31	High
Spaghetti, Buckwheat	1 cup cooked (140g)	42g	45	Low	19	Med.
Spaghetti, Capellini	1 cup cooked (140g)	49g	45	Low	22	High
Spaghetti, Carrot	1 cup cooked (140g)	49g	45	Low	22	High
Spaghetti, Gluten-Free	1 cup cooked (140g)	46g	52	Low	24	High
Spaghetti, Multigrain	1 cup cooked (140g)	46g	40	Low	18	Med.
Spaghetti, Spinach	1 cup cooked (140g)	49g	45	Low	22	High

FOOD	SERVING SIZE	NET CARB (g)	GI VALUE	GI LEVEL	GL VALUE	GL LEVEL
Spaghetti, Squid Ink	1 cup cooked (140g)	49g	45	Low	22	High
Spaghetti, Whole Wheat	1 cup cooked (140g)	45g	37	Low	17	Med.
Spaghetti, Zucchini (Zoodles)	1 cup (120g))	4g	15	Low	1	Low
Spelt	1 cup (194g)	44g	50	Low	24	High
Spelt Pasta	1 cup cooked (140g)	41g	49	Low	19	Med.
Spinach Lasagna	1 cup (240g))	30g	50	Low	12	Med.
Steel-Cut Oats	1 cup cooked (240g)	27g	55	Low	15	Med.
Sun-Dried Tomato Penne	2 ounces (56g)	41g	50	Low	18	Med.
Tapioca Pearl Dry	1 cup (152g)	122g	75	High	43	High
Teff	1 cup (252g)	42g	50	Low	17	Med.
Teff Porridge	1 cup cooked (240g)	29g	75	High	18	Med.
Traditional Lasagna	1 cup (240g))	36g	50		14	Med.
Tricolor Penne	2 ounces (56g)	41g	50		18	Med.
Triticale	1 cup cooked (182g)	40g	50	Low	19	Med.
Triticale Flour Whole-Grain	1 cup (120g)	72g	50	Low	27	High
Udon	1 cup cooked (160g)	52g	55	Low	28	High
Vegetarian Lasagna	1 cup (240g))	25g	50	Low	10	Low

FOOD	SERVING SIZE	NET CARB (g)	GI VALUE	GI LEVEL	GL VALUE	GL LEVEL
Vermicelli	1 cup cooked (140g)	49g	45	Low	22	High
Vermicelli Made From Soybeans	1 cup cooked (150g)	12g	25	Low	5	Low
Wheat Berries	1 cup cooked (198g)	45g	45	Low	20	High
Wheat Bran Crude	1 cup (58g)	20g	45	Low	7	Low
Wheat Durum	1 cup cooked (182g)	48g	50	Low	22	High
Wheat Flour Whole-Grain	1 cup (120g)	84g	65	Med.	36	High
Wheat Germ Crude	1 cup (115g)	39g	45	Low	15	Med.
Wheat Sprouted	1 cup (110g)	31g	50	Low	17	Med.
White Lasagna	1 cup (240g))	20g	50	Low	8	Low
Whole Grain Sorghum Flour	1 cup (125g)	83g	70	High	33	High
Whole Wheat Couscous	1 cup cooked (157g)	33g	55	Low	22	High
Whole Wheat Pasta	1 cup cooked (140g)	49g	45	Low	22	High
Whole Wheat Penne	2 ounces (56g)	39g	37	Low	7	Low

11
HERBS AND SPICES

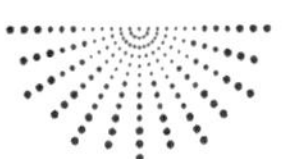

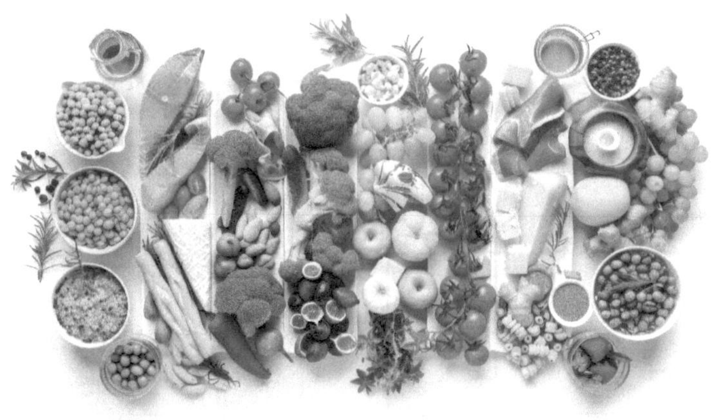

FOOD	SERVING SIZE	NET CARB (g)	GI VALUE	GI LEVEL	GL VALUE	GL LEVEL
Allspice	1 tsp, 2.1 g	1	15	Low	0.2	Low
Anise seeds	1 tsp, 2.1 g	1	0.0	Low	0	Low
Asian chives	1 tbsp, 3 g	1	15	Low	0.2	Low
Basil	1 tsp, 0.7 g	1	70	Low	0.7	Low
Bay leaves	1 tbsp, 1.8 g	0.6	23	Low	0.1	Low
Black cumin	1 tsp, 2.4 g	1	0.0	Low	0	Low
Black pepper	1 tsp, 2.4 g	1	44	Low	0.4	Low
capers	1 tbsp, 8.6 g	0.4	20	Low	0.1	Low
Caraway	1 tbsp, 6.7 g	1	5	Low	0.1	Low
Cardamom	1 tbsp, 5.8 g	1	82	Low	0.8	Low
Celery seed	1 tbsp, 5.8 g	1	32	Low	0.3	Low
Chiles	1 tbsp, 8 g	1	42	Low	0.4	Low
chilli	1 tbsp, 8 g	1	15	Low	0.2	Low

FOOD	SERVING SIZE	NET CARB (g)	GI VALUE	GI LEVEL	GL VALUE	GL LEVEL
Chives	1 tbsp, 2.8 g	1	15	Low	0.2	Low
Cinnamon	1 tbsp, 7.9 g	0.6	70	Low	0.4	Low
Cloves	1 tbsp, 6.6 g	1	87	Low	0.9	Low
Coriander seed	1 tbsp, 5 g	1	33	Low	0.3	Low
Cumin	1 tbsp, 6 g	1.4	0.0	Low	0	Low
Curry Leaves	5 leaves, 2g	1	5	Low	0.1	Low
Curry powder	1 tbsp, 6 g	1	5	Low	0.1	Low
Dill seed	1 tsp, 2.4 g	1	15	Low	0.2	Low
Fennel seeds	1 tbsp, 5.8 g	0	16	Low	0	Low
Fenugreek	1 tbsp, 11.1 g	0.5	25	Low	0.1	Low
Fenugreek Leaves	1 cup, 85 g	3	25	Low	0.8	Low
Five Spice Powder	1 tsp, 2.1 g	1	15	Low	0.2	Low
Garlic chives	2 clove, 6 g	1	15	Low	0.2	Low
Ginger	1 tsp, 2.1 g	1	72	Low	0.7	Low

FOOD	SERVING SIZE	NET CARB (g)	GI VALUE	GI LEVEL	GL VALUE	GL LEVEL
Lemon Balm	1 tsp, 2.1 g	1	15	Low	0.2	Low
Lemongrass	1 cup, 67 g	5.5	45	Low	2.5	Low
Lime Leaves	5 leaves, 2 g	1	32	Low	0.3	Low
Mint	1 tbsp, 3.1 g	1	10	Low	0.1	Low
Mustard Seed	1 tsp, 2 g	1	32	Low	0.3	Low
Nutmeg	1 tsp, 2.4 g	1	46	Low	0.5	Low
Oregano	1 tbsp, 3 g	1	5	Low	0.1	Low
Paprika	1 tsp, 2 g	0.5	15	Low	0.1	Low
Poppy seeds	1 tbsp, 8.8 g	0.4	5	Low	0	Low
Rosemary	1 tbsp, 3.3 g	1	70	Low	0.7	Low
Saffron	1 tsp, 0.7 g	1	70	Low	0.7	Low
Sage	1 tsp, 0.7 g	1	15	Low	0.2	Low
Savory	1 tbsp, 4.4 g	1	16	Low	0.2	Low
Sesame seeds	1 tbsp, 10 g	1	31	Low	0.3	Low

FOOD	SERVING SIZE	NET CARB (g)	GI VALUE	GI LEVEL	GL VALUE	GL LEVEL
Sumac	1 tsp, 2.7 g	1	43	Low	0.4	Low
Summer Savoy	1 tsp, 2.7 g	1	21	Low	0.2	Low
Tarragon	1 tbsp, 1.8g	1	15	Low	0.2	Low
Thyme	1 tbsp, 2.7 g	1	51	Low	0.5	Low
Turmeric	1 tbsp, 6.8 g	1.3	15	Low	0.2	Low
Vanilla	1 tbsp, 4.4 g	1	16	Low	0.2	Low
Wasabi powder	1 tsp, 2.8 g	2	31	Low	0.6	Low
Watercress	1 cup, 34 g	0.5	32	Low	0.2	Low
Wild garlic	1 oz, 28 g	3	11	Low	0.3	Low

12

NUTS & SEEDS

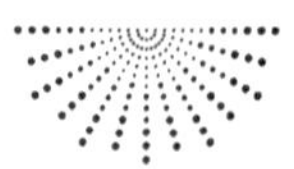

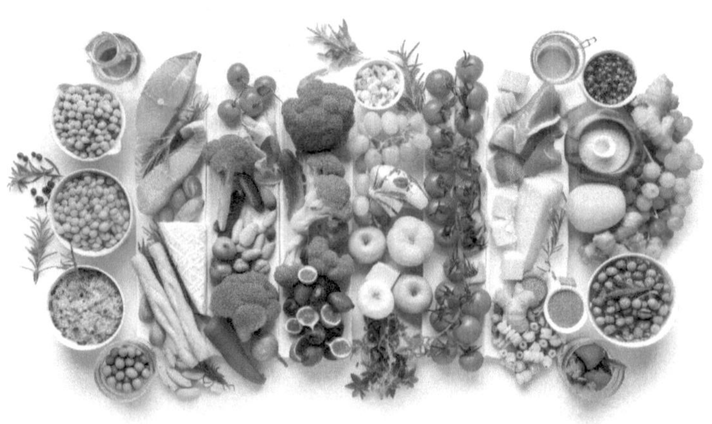

FOOD	SERVING SIZE	NET CARB (g)	GI VALUE	GI LEVEL	GL VALUE	GL LEVEL
Almond Butter	2 tbsp, 32g	3	10	Low	0.3	Low
Almonds Raw/Roasted	1 oz, 28g	2	7	Low	0.2	Low
Brazil Nut Butter	2 tbsp, 32g	2	15	Low	0.3	Low
Brazil nuts Raw/Roasted	1 oz, 28g	1	15	Low	0.2	Low
Butternuts	1 oz, 28g	2	15	Low	0.3	Low
Cashew Butter	2 tbsp, 32g	6	25	Low	1.5	Low
Cashews Raw/Roasted	1 oz, 28g	8	25	Low	2	Low
Chestnuts Boiled	1 oz, 28g	14	60	Med.	8.4	Low
Chestnuts Raw	1 oz, 28g	14	60	Med.	8.4	Low
Chestnuts Roasted	1 oz, 28g	14	60	Med.	8.4	Low
Chestnuts Steamed	1 oz, 28g	14	60	Med.	8.4	Low
Chia Nut Butter	2 tbsp, 32g	2	1	Low	0	Low
Chia Seeds Raw/Roasted	1 oz, 28g	2.2	5	Low	0.1	Low
Fennel seeds	1 oz, 28g	2	5	Low	0.1	Low
Fenugreek seeds	1 oz, 28g	6	15	Low	0.9	Low
Filbert Butter	2 tbsp, 32g	3	0	Low	0	Low
Filberts	1 oz, 28g	2	0	Low	0	Low
Flaxseeds	1 oz, 28g	0	55	Low	0	Low

FOOD	SERVING SIZE	NET CARB (g)	GI VALUE	GI LEVEL	GL VALUE	GL LEVEL
Hazelnut Butter	2 tbsp, 32g	3	15	Low	0.5	Low
Hazelnuts Raw/Roasted	1 oz, 28g	2	15	Low	0.3	Low
Hemp seeds	1 oz, 28g	1	0	Low	0	Low
Macadamia Nut Butter	2 tbsp, 32g	3	15	Low	0.5	Low
Macadamia nuts Raw/Roasted	1 oz, 28g	2	15	Low	0.3	Low
Mustard seeds	1 oz, 28g	2	15	Low	0.3	Low
Peanut Butter	2 tbsp, 32g	6	20	Low	1.2	Low
Peanuts Raw/Roasted	1 oz, 28g	3	14	Low	0.4	Low
Pecan Butter	2 tbsp, 32g	2	0	Low	0	Low
Pecans Raw/Roasted	1 oz, 28g	1	0	Low	0	Low
Pine Nut Oil	1 tbsp, 14g	0	15	Low	0	Low
Pine nuts Raw/Roasted	1 oz, 28g	4	15	Low	0.6	Low
Pistachio Butter	2 tbsp, 32g	4	17	Low	0.6	Low
Pistachios Raw/Roasted	1 oz, 28g	5	15	Low	0.8	Low
Poppy seeds	1 oz, 28g	3	5	Low	0.2	Low
Pumpkin seeds	1 oz, 28g	2	15	Low	0.3	Low
Quinoa seeds	1 oz, 28g	4	53	Low	2.1	Low

FOOD	SERVING SIZE	NET CARB (g)	GI VALUE	GI LEVEL	GL VALUE	GL LEVEL
Sesame seeds	1 oz, 28g	3	35	Low	1.1	Low
Sunflower seeds	1 oz, 28g	3	15	Low	0.5	Low
Tiger nuts	1 oz, 28g	11	51	Low	5.6	Low
Walnut Oil	1 tbsp, 14g	0	0	Low	0	Low
Walnuts Raw/Roasted	1 oz, 28g	1	15	Low	0.2	Low
Watermelon seeds	1 oz, 28g	1	10	Low	0.1	Low

13

VEGETABLES & VEGETABLE PRODUCTS

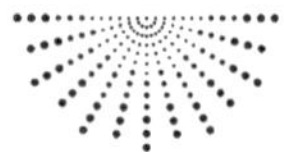

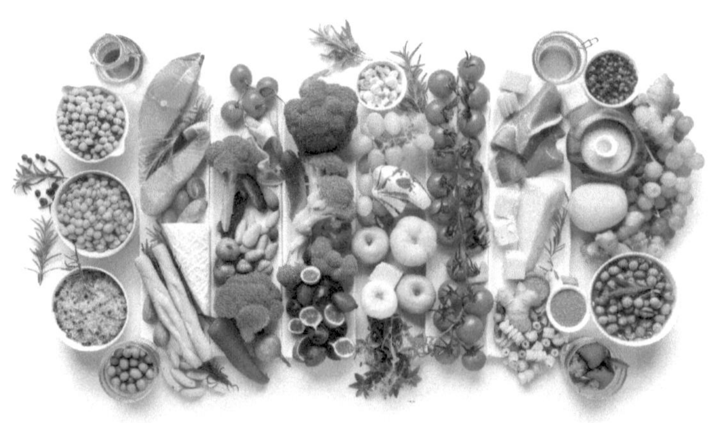

FOOD	SERVING SIZE	NET CARB (g)	GI VALUE	GI LEVEL	GL VALUE	GL LEVEL
Alfalfa Sprouts	1 cup, 33g	0.4	15	Low	1	Low
Amaranth Leaves	1 cup, 132g	5.4	65	Med.	4	Low
Artichoke	1 med., 120g	9	20	Low	3	Low
Artichoke {globe or french), raw	1 med., 120g	4.2	20	Low	4	Low
Artichoke Hearts	1 cup, 168g	12	20	Low	5	Low
Arugula, raw	1 cup, 20g	0.4	30	Low	0	Low
Asparagus	1 cup, 134g	4	15	Low	1	Low
Avocado	½ fruit, 100g	2	15	Low	0	Low
Balsam-pear (bitter gourd), pods, raw	1 cup, 93g	2.3	25	Low	1	Low
Bamboo Shoots	1 cup, 151g	3	15	Low	1	Low
Bean Sprouts	1 cup, 104g	4	30	Low	2	Low
Beet Greens, Raw	1 cup, 144g	3	15	Low	1	Low
Beets, raw	1 cup, 136g	13	69	Med.	5	Low

FOOD	SERVING SIZE	NET CARB (g)	GI VALUE	GI LEVEL	GL VALUE	GL LEVEL
Bell Peppers	1 cup, 149g	6	15	Low	1	Low
Bitter Melon	½ cup, 100g	4	30	Low	3	Low
Bok Choy, Raw	1 cup, 170g	1	15	Low	0	Low
Borage, raw	1 cup, 89g	0.6	20	Low	1	Low
Broccoflower, Raw	1 cup, 100g	3	15	Low	1	Low
Broccoli	1 cup, 156g	6	15	Low	1	Low
Broccoli Raab, raw	1 cup, 40g	0.7	20	Low	1	Low
Broccoli, Chinese, raw	1 cup, 56g	1.8	20	Low	1	Low
Broccoli, leaves, raw	1 cup, 50g	1.4	20	Low	1	Low
Broccoli, stalks, raw	1 cup, 92g	3.3	20	Low	1	Low
Brussels Sprouts, Cooked	1 cup, 156g	8	15	Low	2	Low
Burdock root, raw	1 cup, 116g	14.3	50	Low	7	Low
Butterbur (fuki), raw	1 cup, 55g	1.5	20	Low	1	Low
Butternut Squash	1 cup, 205g	21	51	Low	8	Low

FOOD	SERVING SIZE	NET CARB (g)	GI VALUE	GI LEVEL	GL VALUE	GL LEVEL
Cabbage Green	1 cup, 205g	4	15	Low	1	Low
Cabbage, Chinese (pak-choi), raw	1 cup, 70g	1	20	Low	1	Low
Cabbage, Chinese (pe-tsai), raw	1 cup, 76g	1.2	20	Low	1	Low
Cabbage, raw	1 cup, 89g	3	20	Low	1	Low
Cabbage, red, raw	1 cup, 89g	4	20	Low	1	Low
Cabbage, savoy, raw	1 cup, 70g	2.5	20	Low	1	Low
Cardoon, raw	1 cup, 120g	3.5	20	Low	1	Low
Carrot Greens	1 cup, 25g	1	15	Low	0	Low
Carrots, baby, raw	1 cup, 128g	11.5	54	Low	6	Low
Cassava	½ cup, 110g	39	46	Low	18	Med.
Cauliflower Greens	1 cup, 56g	2	15	Low	1	Low
Celeriac	1 cup, 156g	6	15	Low	1	Low
Celery	1 cup, 101g	2	15	Low	0	Low
Chard, Raw	1 cup, 175g	5	15	Low	1	Low

FOOD	SERVING SIZE	NET CARB (g)	GI VALUE	GI LEVEL	GL VALUE	GL LEVEL
Chayote, Raw	1 cup, 132g	4	15	Low	1	Low
Chicory greens, raw	1 cup, 55g	0.5	20	Low	1	Low
Chicory roots, raw	1 cup, 60g	4	25	Low	1	Low
Chicory, witloof, raw	1 cup, 50g	0.8	20	Low	1	Low
Chives	1 tbsp, 3g	0	15	Low	0	Low
Chrysanthemum leaves, raw	1 cup, 43g	0.6	20	Low	1	Low
Chrysanthemum, garland	1 cup, 20g	1.2	20	Low	1	Low
Collard Greens	1 cup, 190g	5	15	Low	1	Low
Corn, sweet, white, raw	½ cup, 82g	19	60	Med.	11.4	Med.
Corn, sweet, yellow, raw	½ cup, 82g	19	60	Med.	11.4	Med.
Courgette (zucchini baby), raw	1 cup, 127g	3	15	Low	1	Low
Cress, garden, raw	1 cup, 25g	0.7	20	Low	1	Low
Cucumber, peeled, raw	1 cup, 133g	2.5	15	Low	1	Low
Cucumber, with peel, raw	1 cup, 104g	3	15	Low	1	Low

FOOD	SERVING SIZE	NET CARB (g)	GI VALUE	GI LEVEL	GL VALUE	GL LEVEL
Daikon	1 cup, 116g	4	15	Low	1	Low
Dandelion Greens, Raw	1 cup, 55g	3	15	Low	1	Low
Dock, raw	1 cup, 133g	2	20	Low	1	Low
Drumstick leaves, raw	1 cup, 21g	0.5	20	Low	1	Low
Drumstick pods, raw	1 cup, 99g	4	25	Low	2	Low
Edamame Unprepared	½ cup, 75g	8	15	Low	3	Low
Eggplant, Raw	1 cup, 99g	6	15	Low	1	Low
Endive Leaves	1 cup, 40g	1	15	Low	0	Low
Epazote, raw	1 cup, 20g	0.7	20	Low	1	Low
Eppaw, raw	1 cup, 20g	1	20	Low	1	Low
Escarole	1 cup, 75g	3	15	Low	1	Low
Fennel Bulb	1 cup, 87g	5	15	Low	1	Low
Fiddlehead ferns, raw	1 cup, 87g	4	20	Low	1	Low
Fireweed, leaves, raw	1 cup, 35g	1.5	20	Low	1	Low

FOOD	SERVING SIZE	NET CARB (g)	GI VALUE	GI LEVEL	GL VALUE	GL LEVEL
Gourd, dishcloth (towelgourd), raw	1 cup, 86g	2	20	Low	1	Low
Gourd, white-flowered (calabash), raw	1 cup, 116g	3	20	Low	1	Low
Grape leaves	1 cup, 28g	1.5	20	Low	1	Low
Green Onion	1 cup, 100g	4	15	Low	1	Low
Hearts of palm, raw	1 cup, 146g	4	20	Low	1	Low
Hubbard Squash	1 cup, 205g	16	50	Low	6	Low
Jalapeno	1 pepper, 14g	1	15	Low	0	Low
Jerusalem Artichokes	½ cup, 150g	11	50	Low	3	Low
Jicama	1 cup, 120g	6	15	Low	2	Low
Jute, potherb, raw	1 cup, 28g	0.5	20	Low	1	Low
Kale	1 cup, 130g	4	15	Low	1	Low
Kelp	1 cup, 76g	1	15	Low	0	Low
Kohlrabi	1 cup, 135g	8	15	Low	2	Low

FOOD	SERVING SIZE	NET CARB (g)	GI VALUE	GI LEVEL	GL VALUE	GL LEVEL
Lambsquarters, raw	1 cup, 28g	1	20	Low	1	Low
Leek Leaves	1 cup, 72g	4	15	Low	1	Low
Lemon grass (citronella), raw	1 tbsp, 6g	0.4	20	Low	1	Low
Lettuce, green leaf, raw	1 cup, 36g	1	15	Low	1	Low
Lettuce, iceberg (includes crisphead types), raw	1 cup, 72g	1	15	Low	1	Low
Lettuce, red leaf, raw	1 cup, 28g	0.7	15	Low	1	Low
Lettuce, Romaine	1 cup, 72g	1	15	Low	0	Low
Lotus Root	1 cup, 120g	16	60	Med.	7	Low
Malabar spinach (Vine), raw	1 cup, 44g	0.8	20	Low	1	Low
Mountain yam, hawaii, raw	½ cup, 82g	18	58	Med.	11	Med.
Mushroom	1 cup, 70g	2	15	Low	0	Low
Mushrooms (Portobello, Shiitake, etc.)	1 cup, 86g	2	15	Low	0	Low
Mustard spinach, raw	1 cup, 56g	1.5	20	Low	1	Low
Napa Cabbage	1 cup, 109g	3	15	Low	1	Low

FOOD	SERVING SIZE	NET CARB (g)	GI VALUE	GI LEVEL	GL VALUE	GL LEVEL
New Zealand spinach, raw	1 cup, 56g	1	20	Low	1	Low
Nopales	1 cup, 86g	3	15	Low	1	Low
Okra	1 cup, 100g	4	15	Low	1	Low
Olives, Black	1 ounce, 28g	1	15	Low	0	Low
Olives, Green	1 ounce, 28g	1	15	Low	0	Low
Onions, spring or scallions, raw	1 cup, 100g	6	35	Low	3	Low
Onions, sweet, raw	1 cup, 160g	14	35	Low	5	Low
Onions, welsh, raw	1 cup, 100g	7	35	Low	3	Low
Parsley	1 tbsp, 3g	0	15	Low	0	Low
Parsnip	½ cup, 78g	12	52	Low	6	Low
Peppers, hot chili, green, raw	1 pepper, 14g	1	35	Low	1	Low
Peppers, hot chili, red, raw	1 pepper, 45g	2	35	Low	1	Low
Peppers, Hungarian, raw	1 cup, 125g	5	20	Low	1	Low

FOOD	SERVING SIZE	NET CARB (g)	GI VALUE	GI LEVEL	GL VALUE	GL LEVEL
Peppers, jalapeno, raw	1 pepper, 14g	0.6	35	Low	1	Low
Peppers, serrano, raw	1 pepper, 18g	1	35	Low	1	Low
Peppers, sweet, green, raw	1 cup, 149g	6	20	Low	2	Low
Peppers, sweet, red, raw	1 cup, 149g	6	20	Low	2	Low
Peppers, sweet, yellow, raw	1 cup, 149g	6	20	Low	2	Low
Potato, Cooked	½ cup, 105g	15	78	High	11	Low
Potatoes, flesh and skin, raw	1 med., 213g	33	65	Med.	18	Med.
Pumpkin leaves, raw	1 cup, 33g	0.6	20	Low	1	Low
Pumpkin, mashed	1 cup, 245g	9.3	78	High	7.5	Low
Purslane, raw	1 cup, 43g	0.7	20	Low	1	Low
Radicchio	1 cup, 40g	1	15	Low	0	Low
Radish	1 cup, 116g	2	15	Low	0	Low
Rhubarb	1 cup, 122g	5	15	Low	1	Low

FOOD	SERVING SIZE	NET CARB (g)	GI VALUE	GI LEVEL	GL VALUE	GL LEVEL
Rutabaga	½ cup, 85g	8	72	High	5	Low
Salsify, raw	1 cup, 133g	8	35	Low	3	Low
Seaweed, agar, raw	1 cup, 40g	1	20	Low	1	Low
Seaweed, irishmoss, raw	1 cup, 40g	2	20	Low	1	Low
Seaweed, kelp, raw	1 cup, 36g	1	20	Low	1	Low
Seaweed, laver, raw	1 cup, 25g	1	20	Low	1	Low
Seaweed, spirulina, raw	1 tbsp, 7g	0.3	20	Low	1	Low
Seaweed, wakame, raw	1 cup, 10g	0.5	20	Low	1	Low
Sesbania flower, raw	1 cup, 25g	1	20	Low	1	Low
Shallot	1 tbsp, 10g	2	15	Low	0.3	Low
Sorrel	1 cup, 29g	1	15	Low	0	Low
Spinach	1 cup, 180g	4	15	Low	0.6	Low
Squash Acorn	½ cup, 102g	15	75	High	7.5	Low
Squash Butternut	½ cup, 102g	21	51	Low	8	Low

FOOD	SERVING SIZE	NET CARB (g)	GI VALUE	GI LEVEL	GL VALUE	GL LEVEL
Squash Spaghetti	1 cup, 155g	7	15	Low	1	Low
Sweet potato leaves, raw	1 cup, 28g	1	20	Low	1	Low
Sweet Potato, Boiled	1 serv., 75g	15	50	Low	7.5	Low
Sweet Potato, Roasted	1 serv., 75g	15	88	High	13.2	Low
Swiss Chard	1 cup, 175g	4	15	Low	1	Low
Taro leaves, raw	1 cup, 28g	1	20	Low	1	Low
Taro shoots, raw	1 cup, 84g	2	20	Low	1	Low
Taro, Tahitian, raw	½ cup, 104g	12.5	55	Low	9	Low
Tomatillo	1 cup, 132g	4	15	Low	1	Low
Tomato, chopped	1 cup, 180g	5	15	Low	1	Low
Turnip	1 cup, 156g	8	62	Med.	4	Low
Waterchestnuts, chinese, raw	1 cup, 150g	24	60	Med.	9	Low
Watercress	1 cup, 34g	0	15	Low	0	Low
Yam, boiled	1 cup, 136 g	37	51	Low	18.9	Med.

FOOD	SERVING SIZE	NET CARB (g)	GI VALUE	GI LEVEL	GL VALUE	GL LEVEL
Yam, fried	1 cup, 136 g	37	59	Med.	21.2	High
Yam, roasted	1 cup, 136 g	37	51	Low	18.9	Med.
Zucchini	1 cup, 124g	6	15	Low	2	Low

BIBLIOGRAPHY/REFERENCES

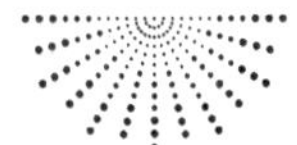

American Diabetes Association (2011). “Diagnosis and classification of diabetes mellitus.” https://doi.org/10.2337/dc11-S062

Astrup (2005). "The role of dietary fat in obesity" https://doi.org/10.1055/s-2005-871740

Atkinson et al. (2014). "Type 1 diabetes." https://doi.org/10.1016/S0140-6736(13)60591-7

Beasley, Wylie-Rosett (2013)."The role of dietary proteins among persons with diabetes." https://doi.org/10.1007/s11883-013-0348-2

Bjørgaas (2000). “Hypoglycemia--a dreaded complication of diabetes.” https://pubmed.ncbi.nlm.nih.gov/11475234/

Blaak et al. (2021). "Carbohydrates: Separating fact from fiction." https://doi.org/10.1016/j.atherosclerosis.2021.03.025

Bornet et al. (1997). "Glycemic index concept and metabolic diseases." https://doi.org/10.1016/s0141-8130(97)00066-4

Brennan (2005). "Dietary fibre, glycemic response, and diabetes." https://doi.org/10.1002/mnfr.200500025

Campos et al. (2022) "Importance of Carbohydrate Quality: What Does It Mean and How to Measure It?" https://doi.org/10.1093/jn/nxac039

Chatterjee et al. (2017). "Type 2 diabetes." https://doi.org/10.1016/S0140-6736(17)30058-2

Chester et al. (2019). "The effects of popular diets on type 2 diabetes management." https://doi.org/10.1002/dmrr.3188

Clemente-Suárez et al. (2022). "The Burden of Carbohydrates in Health and Disease" https://doi.org/10.3390/nu14183809

Davies et al., (2018). "Management of Hyperglycemia in Type 2 Diabetes." https://doi.org/10.2337/dci18-0033

Davis, Wylie-Rosett (2008). "Death to carbohydrate counting?" https://doi.org/10.2337/dc08-0807

DeFronzo et al (2015). "Type 2 diabetes mellitus." https://doi.org/10.1038/nrdp.2015.19

Deshpande et al. (2008). "Epidemiology of diabetes and diabetes-related complications." https://doi.org/10.2522/ptj.20080020

DiMeglio et al., (2018). "Type 1 diabetes." https://doi.org/10.1016/S0140-6736(18)31320-5

E. Lee (2019). Intake of Fruits for Diabetics: Why and How Much? https://doi.org/10.4093/jkd.2019.20.2.106

Emadian et al. (2015). "The effect of macronutrients on glycemic control." https://doi.org/10.1017/S0007114515003475

Esposito et al. (2009) " Which diet is best for diabetes?" https://doi.org/10.1007/s00125-009-1292-0

Fan (2024). "Primordial Drivers of Diabetes Heart Disease" https://doi.org/10.4093/dmj.2023.0110

Fletche (2002). "Risk factors for type 2 diabetes mellitus." https://doi.org/10.1097/00005082-200201000-00003

Flint et al. (2005)"The use of glycemic index tables to predict glycemic index of breakfast meals." https://doi.org/10.1079/bjn20041424

Forbes et al. (2013). "Mechanisms of Diabetic Complications." https://doi.org/10.1152/physrev.00045.2011

Fresh fruit consumption in relation to incident diabetes and diabetic vascular complications. https://doi.org/10.1371/journal.pmed.1002279

Frontoni et al. (2005). Papamichou et al. (2019)."Dietary patterns and management of type 2 diabetes" https://doi.org/10.1016/j.numecd.2019.02.004

Geekie et al. (1986)."Acceptability of high-fibre diets in diabetic patients." https://doi.org/10.1111/j.1464-5491.1986.tb00710.x.

Giugliano et al. (2018). "More sugar? No, thank you! The elusive nature of low carb diets."https://doi.org/10.1007/s12020-018-1580-x

Greenbaum (2002). “Insulin resistance in type 1 diabetes.” https://doi.org/10.1002/dmrr.291

Gregg, Sattar (2016). "Global epidemiology and prevention of type 2 diabetes and its complications." https://doi.org/10.1038/nrendo.2015.223

Großkopf, Simm (2024). "Carbohydrates in nutrition: friend or foe?" https://doi.org/10.1007/s00391-020-01726-1

Hamdy, Horton (2011)."Protein content in diabetes nutrition plan." https://doi.org/10.1007/s11892-010-0171-x

Harding et al. (2019). “Global trends in diabetes complications” https://doi.org/10.1007/s00125-018-4711-2

J. Dias, S. Imai (2017). Vegetables Consumption and its Benefits on Diabetes. https://doi.org/10.6000/1929-5634.2017.06.01.1

Jenkins et al. (1981). "Glycemic index of foods: a physiological basis for carbohydrate exchange." https://doi.org/10.1093/ajcn/34.3.362

Kalra et al. (2013). “Hypoglycemia: The neglected complication.” https://doi.org/10.4103/2230-8210.117219

Khazrai et al. (2014) "Effect of diet on type 2 diabetes mellitus: a review." https://doi.org/10.1002/dmrr.2515

Kirkpatrick et al. (2022). "How low should one go in reducing carbohydrate?" https://doi.org/10.1016/j.jacl.2022.10.007

Kolarić et al. (2022). “Chronic Complications of Diabetes and Quality of Life.” https://doi.org/10.20471/acc.2022.61.03.18

Lamothe et al. (2017). "The scientific basis for healthful carbohydrate profile." https://doi.org/10.1080/10408398.2017.1392287

Liston et al. (2017). “Beta-Cell Fragility As a Common Underlying Risk Factor in Type 1 and Type 2 Diabetes.” https://doi.org/10.1016/j.molmed.2016.12.005

Looker et al. (2012). "Diabetic retinopathy at diagnosis of type 2 diabetes" https://doi.org/10.1007/s00125-012-2595-3

Malone (2019). “Does obesity cause type 2 diabetes mellitus (T2DM)? Or is it the opposite?.” https://doi.org/10.1111/pedi.12787

Ndisang et al. (2017). “Insulin Resistance, Type 1 and Type 2 Diabetes, and Related Complications 2017.” https://doi.org/10.1155/2017/1478294

Neuhouser (2019)."The importance of healthy dietary patterns in chronic disease prevention." https://doi.org/10.1016/j.nutres.2018.06.002

Nicholas et al. (2021). "Restricting carbohydrates and calories in the treatment of type 2 diabetes." https://doi.org/10.1017/10.1017/jns.2021.67

Olsson et al. (2021). "Associations of carbohydrates and carbohydrate-rich foods with incidence of type 2 diabetes." https://doi.org/10.1017/S0007114520005140

Papamichou et al. (2019)."Dietary patterns and management of type 2 diabetes" https://doi.org/10.1016/j.numecd.2019.02.004

Petersmann et al. (2019). "Definition, Classification and Diagnosis of Diabetes Mellitus." https://doi.org/10.1055/a-1018-9078

Rivellese et al. (2012). "Dietary carbohydrates for diabetics." https://doi.org/10.1007/s11883-012-0278-4

Sawyer, Gale (2009). "Diet, delusion and diabetes." https://doi.org/10.1007/s00125-008-1203-9

Seckold et al. (2018)"The ups and downs of low-carbohydrate diets in the management of Type 1 diabetes" https://doi.org/10.1111/dme.13845

Shkembi et al., 2023. Glycemic Responses of Milk and Plant." https://www.ncbi.nlm.nih.gov/pmc/articles/PMC9914410/

Slavin JL, Lloyd B. (2012). "Health Benefits of fruits and vegetables." https://doi.org/10.3945/an

Slavin, Carlson (2014). "Carbohydrates" https://doi.org/10.3945/an.114.006163

Solis-Herrera et al. (2021). "Pathogenesis of Type 2 Diabetes Mellitus." https://www.ncbi.nlm.nih.gov/books/NBK279115/

Taylor (2013). "Type 2 diabetes: etiology and reversibility." https://doi.org/10.2337/dc12-1805.

Vasiljevic et al. (2020). "The making of insulin in health and disease." https://doi.org/10.1007/s00125-020-05192-7

Vinik, Jenkins (1988) "Dietary fiber in management of diabetes." https://doi.org/10.2337/diacare.11.2.160

Widanagamage et al. (2009). "Carbohydrate-rich foods: glycemic index and the effect of constituent macronutrients." https://doi.org/10.1080/09637480902849195.

Wilcox (2005). "Insulin and insulin resistance." https://www.ncbi.nlm.nih.gov/pmc/articles/PMC1204764/

Wolever et al. (1992). "Beneficial effect of a low glycemic index diet in type 2 diabetes." https://doi.org/10.1111/j.1464-5491.1992.tb01816.x

Workeneh, Mitch (2013)."High-protein diet in diabetic nephropathy: what is really safe?" https://doi.org/10.3945/ajcn.113.067223

Yen, et al. (2022). “Increased vegetable intake improves glycemic control in adults with type 2 diabetes mellitus.” https://doi.org/10.2337/dc11-S062

Zhou et al. (2022). "Gut Microbiota: An Important Player in Type 2 Diabetes Mellitus." https://doi.org/10.3389/fcimb.2022.834485

HEALTH AND NUTRITION WEBSITES

- Centers for Disease Control and Prevention: https://www.cdc.gov/healthyweight
- Fruits and Vegetables Matter: https://www.fruitsandveggiesmatter.gov
- Cooking Light: https://www.cookinglight.com
- Nutrition.gov: https://www.nutrition.gov
- Hormone Foundation: https://www.hormone.org
- American Diabetes Association: https://www.diabetes.org
- American Heart Association: https://www.americanheart.org
- National Institute on Aging: https://www.nia.nih.gov
- National Institutes of Health: http://health.nih.gov
- National Kidney Disease Education Program | NIDDK: https://www.niddk.nih.gov/health-information/community-health-outreach/information-clearinghouses/nkdep
- American Kidney Fund (AKF): https://www.kidneyfund.org/
- The National Institute of Diabetes and Digestive and Kidney Diseases (NIDDK): https://www.niddk.nih.gov/health-information/kidney-disease

ABOUT THE AUTHOR

Dr. H. Maher" is a joint pen name under which Dr. Y. Naitlho, PharmD (Doctor of Pharmacy), and H. Naitlho, MEng (ISAE-SUPAERO), MEng (École de l'Air et de l'Espace), Advanced MSc (Paul Sabatier University), and Executive MBA, co-write books.

Dr. Y. Naitlho, PharmD, brings over 25 years of experience in pharmacy practice, with a special emphasis on nutrition, healthy eating, and writing. He obtained his Doctor of Pharmacy degree from the Perm State Pharmaceutical Academy in 1998. Dr. Y. Naitlho is notably active within the healthcare community, particularly through his community pharmacy. He, along with his pharmacy team, spearheads patient education initiatives, providing medication counseling, printed educational materials, and advice on dietary regulation, exercise, and lifestyle adjustments for patients managing chronic diseases such as diabetes, hypertension, heart disease, and kidney disorders.

Additionally, Dr. Y. Naitlho participates in humanitarian campaigns in collaboration with multidisciplinary healthcare professionals, including endocrinologists, cardiologists, ophthalmologists, and nephrologists. This joint effort is designed to deliver comprehensive support to those in need, ensuring they receive the most effective and optimal care available.

H. Naitlho possesses over 30 years of experience in engineering, operations, project management, as well as in scientific and engineering research. He is an established author of several books on business management and a co-author of a vast array of publications on food science, human nutrition, food engineering, and applied nutrition. H. Naitlho earned a Master of Systems Engineering from the École Nationale Supérieure d'Aéronautique et de l'Espace (ISAE-SUPAERO), a Master in Aeronautical Systems Engineering from the French Air and Space Force Academy, an Advanced Master in Automatics from Paul Sabatier University, and an additional Master's degree in Mechanical Engineering from Aix Marseille University, alongside an Executive MBA from Laureate International Universities. His engineering mindset and scientific rigor enhance their collaborative work, demonstrating a meticulous approach to refining ideas, analyzing data, and ensuring consistency and attention to detail in their writing projects.

Together, Dr. Y. Naitlho and H. Naitlho share a profound commitment to assisting individuals with diabetes, chronic kidney disease (CKD), and hypertension in leading healthier, more satisfying lives through informed food choices and customized meal plans. They are dedicated to keeping abreast of the latest research and nutritional guidelines to furnish their readers with accurate, dependable, and actionable information. Their combined efforts culminate in books that empower those with these health conditions to take control of their health and savor a diverse, nutritious diet.